Lady With A Lamp:
An Untold Story of Florence Nightingale

"With veracious historic grit and not-ever so proper Victorian perspective, Lady with a Lamp depicts Florence Nightingale's Crimean War experiences through the eyes of the small-minded and blood-guilty characters surrounding her."

Diane L. LaSala
Director of Lady with a Lamp

"Neary's Lady With A Lamp lights our way beyond the legendary Florence Nightingale to the human being beneath, and illuminates the darker corners of her soul, unexplored by the public."

Lewayne L. White
President, Iowa Scriptwriters Alliance

Lady With A Lamp:
An Untold Story of
Florence Nightingale

by

Marina Julia Neary

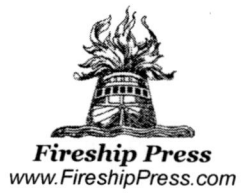

Fireship Press
www.FireshipPress.com

LADY WITH A LAMP: An Untold Story of Florence Nightingale
- Copyright © 2009 by Marina Julia Neary

ISBN-13: 978-1-934757-98-7
ISBN-10: 1-934757-98-5

BISAC Subject Headings:
    DRA003000   DRAMA / English, Irish, Scottish, Welsh
    MED058000   MEDICAL / Nursing / General
    MED039000   MEDICAL / History

We would like to thank Richard Megenis for permission to use his excellent photos of the premier performance of this play.

Address all correspondence to:
Fireship Press, LLC
P.O. Box 68412
Tucson, AZ 85737

Or visit our website at:
www.FireshipPress.com

1.0

Contents

About the Play

"Lady with a Lamp" premiered in Greenwich, CT in October, 2009 as a theatrical benefit for The Wyatt Foundation, a group that was created for the purpose of educating the public about muscular dystrophy. As the author and executive producer, I thought it would be appropriate to tie the play with a medically-oriented non-profit given the altruistic reputation of the title heroine. Even though the play is set in 1854, it touches upon certain issues that are, sadly, still relevant today—medical malpractice, controversial military campaigns, and political corruption.

The play emerged as a sequel to my previous tragicomedy "Hugo in London" (a theatrical spinoff of *Wynfield's Kingdom*) that premiered in 2008 and was recently acquired by Heuer Publishing. I should note that my choice of actors for "Lady with a Lamp" predates the actual writing of the script. The characters of Bennett and Martin were written with two actors in mind. David Thomas McLaine (Bennett) and Joseph Saulnier (Martin) portrayed young aristocrats in the Parliament scene in "Hugo." Intrigued by their wide range of mannerisms and expressions, I wanted to see them in more challenging and fleshed out roles that would allow them to engage their abilities more fully. Connecticut is gradually gaining a national reputation as a center for exceptional theatrical talent, and I prefer to use local actors when possible.

Joseph Saulnier is a martial arts champion and, consequently, channels his energy in a very controlled manner. Fit, composed and disciplined in real life, he needed to step out of his body to embrace the role of a disoriented, ranting amputee. Being of French, Italian and Native American descent, Joseph has a dark complexion and pronounced masculine features, all of which high-

i

light the irony of his character being crippled and demeaned, fighting for the remains of his dignity.

David Thomas McLaine, with his tangerine hair, sapphire eyes and boyish features, exudes mischievous vigor. He speaks in a high, melodic tenor, which would not be out of place in an Anglican boy choir. Atrocious acts coming from someone who looks like a vaudeville villain are not shocking to the audience. An angel-faced sadist, however, is far more sinister. Having such contrasting appearances, David and Joseph complement each other as stage enemies.

The role of Rebecca, the incompetent young nurse who becomes their bone of contention, was played by *Angessa Hughmanick*, an accomplished ballerina and choreographer. Like Joseph, she had to step out of her graceful, toned body to become a clumsy, skittish creature. For the audience, she provided a mixture of beauty and much-needed comic relief.

There is another pair of rivals in the play—Lord Cardigan and his immediate superior and brother-in-law Lord Lucan. In the aftermath of the disastrous charge of the Light Brigade, the two incurably arrogant men engage in a juvenile match of finger-pointing before the cabin boy played by *Alex Mair*.

Michael Hogan, who played the title role in "Hugo," delivered a deliciously grotesque performance as Cardigan, an extravagant drunk.

Walt Neary, who grew up on BBC productions, finally realized his dream of portraying a corrupt British general. Pale, angular and effortlessly slender like the historical Lucan, he made a gallant villain.

Philip Gardiner, the main instigator of the sequel, continued in his role as Tom Grant, a dethroned, opium-trading sociopath, a broken-down physical and intellectual giant haunted by the ghosts of his departed foster children. With the exquisite mastery of a stage veteran, Philip communicated the astonishment of a man who, in a state of penitentiary exile, is suddenly swept up by a whirlwind of political intrigue, temptation and love.

Tall and broad-shouldered, Philip emphasized the outward delicacy of his co-star *Marta Coppola*, whose porcelain skin, elegant profile and enormous hazel eyes have solicited much admiration from artists, photographers and producers. After portraying a delusional young heiress endowed with some of the least commendable female traits, Marta returns to the stage as Florence Nightingale. As a writer, I did not attempt an historically exhaustive portrayal of the heroine. A slogan-spouting cardboard saint would probably not endear herself to an audience very much. My goal was to present Florence as a real woman with an ego and libido, a woman who was not afraid of becoming a black sheep in her own family, or making enemies. Having known Marta since the age of fifteen, I knew that she would do this role justice.

I would like to extend gratitude to *George McGarvey*, an Emmy-winning set designer who had generously volunteered his services for the project. The yacht and the hospital were constructed side by side on stage to symbolize the two parallel worlds of the English army—one of the privileged generals and the other of the nameless, dispensable soldiers.

And above all, special thanks to the director *Diane LaSala*, whose dedication and meticulous analysis of the script took the project to new heights.

My gratitude goes out to the entire cast of "Lady with a Lamp" for having brought this play to life so beautifully.

Florence Nightingale - Marta Coppola
Thomas Grant - Philip Gardiner
Timothy Bennett - David Thomas McLaine
Rebecca Prior - Angessa Hughmanick
James Martin - Joseph Saulnier
Lord Cardigan - Michael Hogan
Lord Lucan - Walt Neary
Cabin Boy - Alex Mair

Director - Diane LaSala
Set Design by George McGarvey
Photos by Richard Megenis.

Synopsis

Crimea, 1854: Having botched the Charge of the Light Brigade, Lord Cardigan is hiding on his yacht, drinking himself into stupor. On the shore, at the hospital corps, a mutiny is brewing. Egotistic doctors, brutish surgeons and skittish nurses wage mind wars against each other amidst filth and chaos.

Florence Nightingale, the legendary "Lady with a Lamp" – a saint to her patients and a frigid spinster to her colleagues – finds solace in the company of Tom Grant, a haggard physician with a sinister reputation. Trading grim jokes and scientific facts, the two develop a cerebral romance that promises to mark a new era for English medicine. Inevitably, Tom's semi-criminal past surfaces, throwing him in the political crossfire between Cardigan and Lucan.

In a luxurious stateroom, in the presence of England's most corrupt general, Tom receives an offer no sane man could refuse – a life of prestige and prosperity on the condition is that he must break the Hippocratic Oath and permanently defame another man. What is one more sin to a soul that is already beyond salvation? Above all, what does England's most virtuous woman have to say about her lover's dilemma?

Inspired by historical events, this play is a work of speculative fiction, a sequel to the previous tragicomedy "Hugo in London."

Characters

FLORENCE Nightingale (mid 30s) – the Lady with the Lamp, a nurse of upper-class origin, a slender pale brunette, inconspicuously beautiful, unsentimental, somewhat abrasive, educated above other women, prefers the company of powerful men

GRANT, THOMAS (late 40s) – a weary doctor with a sinister past, Florence's friend and love interest, a broken down physical and intellectual giant

BENNETT, Timothy (early 20s) – a surgeon under Dr. Grant's command, insubordinate, maniacal, with sadistic inclinations, a clean-cut buttoned-down butcher

REBECCA Prior (late teens - early 20s) – a young nurse, beautiful but inarticulate and skittish, prone to contributing to conflicts, becomes the object of Bennett's lust

MARTIN, JAMES (early-mid 20s) – a wounded soldier with a criminal past, hates Bennett whom he blames for the loss of his hand, develops a filial attachment to Florence and a chivalrous infatuation with Rebecca

CARDIGAN, Lord James (James Thomas Brudenell, 7th Earl of Cardigan) (50s) – an incompetent British general, arrogant in public, cowardly in private, tries to put the blame for a botched campaign on Lucan

LUCAN, Lord George (George Charles Bingham, 3rd Earl of Lucan) (50s) – Cardigan's direct commander and brother-in-law, condescending, invincible in his own eyes, scandalous and insensitive

Scene 1

A surgical tent at a field hospital. Half-conscious wounded soldiers are spread over the benches, their limbs wrapped in dirty rags. Rebecca Prior, a young nurse, is sobbing hysterically into a towel. Florence Nightingale is standing over her, unperturbed. Mr. Bennett is pacing behind Rebecca, fuming.

BENNETT (*throws his arms up*): This is preposterous!

REBECCA (*lifts her head*): I'm so dreadfully sorry...

BENNETT: It isn't my forgiveness that you should be begging. Apologize to Private Martin, who had to witness your tantrum from the comfort of the surgical table.

REBECCA: It's that... It's that I've never seen so much blood before.

BENNETT: What did you expect, Miss Prior – a parish outing, a tea ceremony, perhaps? So much for being a butcher's daughter!

Rebecca rubs the bridge of her nose, disoriented.

REBECCA: Miss Nightingale, what happened in there?

BENNETT (*pauses and hovers over Rebecca*): Perhaps, *I* should refresh your memory. You vomited into the surgical tray and dropped it on the floor. I was forced to finish the amputation unassisted.

1

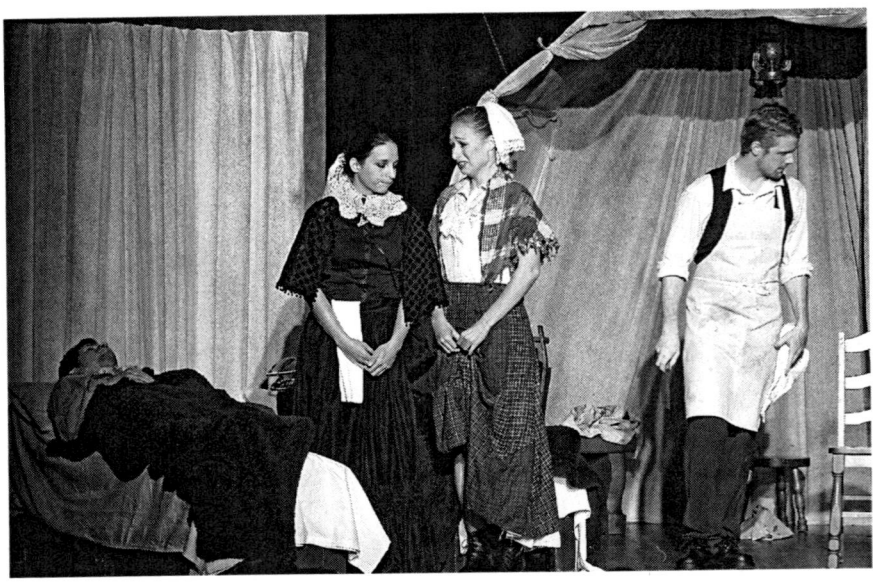

Rebecca gasps into the towel and has another sobbing fit. Florence squeezes Rebecca's head and makes her turn towards Bennett.

FLORENCE: Now, look Mr. Bennett in the eye and promise him in a steady voice that this shall never be repeated.

BENNETT (*to Rebecca*): You can bet your sweet life it won't! You are not to come near the surgical tent ever again. Do you hear me?

Rebecca mumbles indistinctly.

BENNETT: You'll be on the first ship back to England, where you can resume rationing gruel at a workhouse!

FLORENCE (*hastily*): That won't be necessary. If I send every incompetent nurse home, I won't have any hands left. There's a fitting occupation for everyone. I shall put Rebecca in charge of sanitizing the instruments and boiling the laundry. You start with your soiled linens. Remember to soak the blood out with cold water before boiling.

2

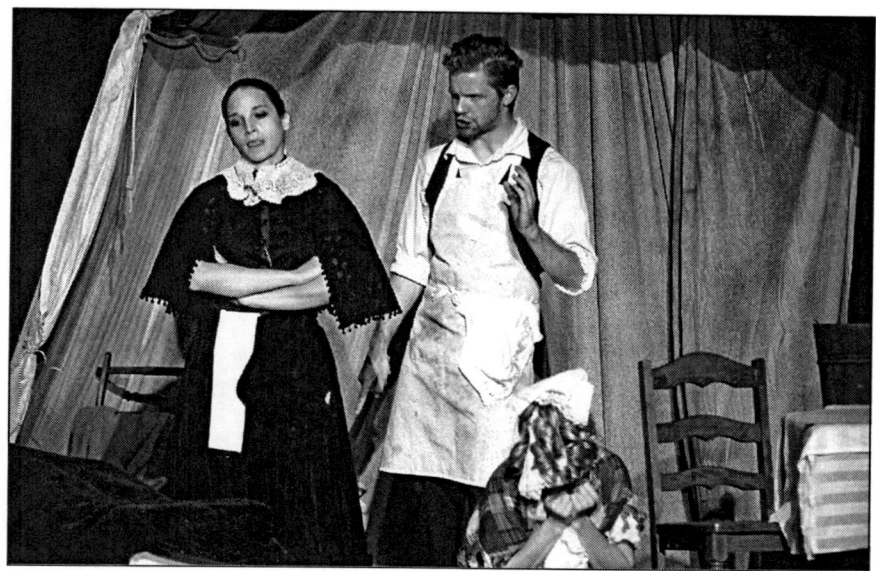

Rebecca nods, pulls her head into her shoulders, picks up the linens timidly and exits. Florence inhales and shakes her head. Bennett wipes his bloody saw nonchalantly and prepares to leave.

FLORENCE: Mr. Bennett, I marvel at the pliancy of your conscience. Taking your personal embarrassment out on a creature like Becky Prior – how convenient!

BENNETT (*coldly*): Miss Nightingale, I don't have the faintest...

FLORENCE (*takes a step forward*): Come now, we both know why you lashed out at Rebecca. Naturally, you are infuriated by your own mistake.

BENNETT (*insulted*): What mistake?

FLORENCE (*gestures towards the surgical tent*): The loss of Private Martin's hand. Had you followed my instructions for cleaning and dressing the wound, the infection would not have spread, and gangrene would not have developed. There would've been no need for such... terminal surgical measures.

BENNETT: I shan't continue this conversation with you.

3

FLORENCE: Very well, then you shall have it with your superiors! I'm certain that Dr. Grant will have something to say regarding this matter. Your imaginary crown won't tarnish if you would heed my advice from time to time. Young man...

BENNETT (*raises his voice*): It's Mr. Bennett to you! I address you by your surname, so please, extend the same courtesy to me. I would be most grateful if you did not project your unused maternal sentiments onto me.

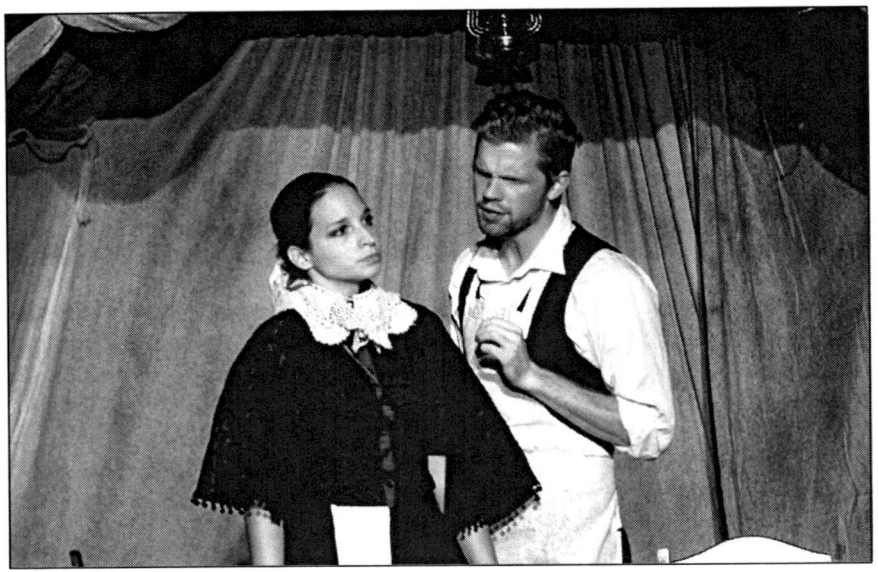

FLORENCE: Rest assured, Mr. Bennett, the good Lord spared me such sentiments. I've been endowed with more practical talents, such as speaking candidly, especially in the face of blatant malpractice and negligence. Crippled soldiers are of no use to England. If you continue to butcher them—

BENNETT (*with sinister softness*): Miss Nightingale, I worry about your well-being. The whites of your eyes are turning quite scarlet. So much righteous anger will do you no good. You recall that you've already suffered one emotional collapse. (*Squints maliciously*) And do not let chloroform go to your brain.

Bennett salutes Florence mockingly and leaves.

4

Scene 2

Florence rubs her temples, breathing unevenly, trying to harness her anger, then sits down on the bench vacated by Rebecca and pulls out a letter from under her blouse, fans herself with it.

FLORENCE (*mutters to herself*): You better start reading my letters, Sidney. What sort of people have you sent here? The nurses dread the sight of blood, and the surgeons like it a bit too much. How am I to establish a hospital?

A coarse cough is heard. Enters Dr. Grant, rolling down the sleeves of his shirt that is stained with dried blood and dirt.

FLORENCE (*savors the sound of coughing*): I hear hundreds of coughs every day, but yours has a distinctive low-pitched undertone that reminds me of...

GRANT: A bear's growl? (*Chuckles tiredly*) After nightfall my ursine nature emerges. Did I miss a mutiny?

Grant goes to check on the patient

FLORENCE: Some of our colleagues take too much pleasure in their profession.

GRANT: Dare I guess: Timmy Bennett delivering another tirade?

FLORENCE: A perfect tyrant at age twenty-two! Imagine, being so young?

GRANT: What would I know about such things? I've been forty-nine my entire life.

FLORENCE: Rest assured, Dr. Grant, at this pace, I'm not far behind you.

Grant examines Martin and realizes that the whole hand is missing.

GRANT (*mumbles under his breath*): Damn that scrawny butcher... He took the whole hand!

FLORENCE: Who sent him here? He was just a barber from Manchester. I wonder how many customers he slashed in his life. This is what infuriates me. People come here because they have failed at everything else.

Florence's eyes widen.

FLORENCE: A rat! I won't have you infecting my patients, you nasty vermin.

Grant turns around. Florence grabs a broom and chases the rat across the floor, corners and beats it. When Florence holds the rat, she holds it up by the tail.

GRANT: Is this your heroic deed for the day, Miss Nightingale?

FLORENCE: This, Dr. Grant, is material evidence that I shall enclose with my next parcel to England.

GRANT: Save the rat for the next time we run out of provisions. I'm not joking.

Florence discards the rat and wipes her hands.

FLORENCE: I'm still waiting for dressing gauze to be delivered. Soon I will have to tear strips from the hem of my skirt to bandage wounds.

GRANT: If it's any consolation, I have an audience with Cardigan tomorrow. I have no idea why he summoned me, but I'll be sure to plead on your behalf.

FLORENCE: With Lord Cardigan? I wouldn't let my hopes soar.

GRANT: At least I'll see the interior of his infamous yacht. If I'm lucky, I'll catch a whiff of his brandy. It's been a long time since I smelled quality spirits.

FLORENCE: I honestly don't know how much longer I can hold down the fort. The hospital looks like a butchery, even after all my efforts to create a civilized medical establishment. I waste too much time writing letters that make no difference at all.

She sits down on the bench, exhausted.

GRANT: When was the last time you slept?

Their hands brush. Florence notices that Grant's hands are hot and frowns.

FLORENCE: Good God... Have you been laying hot bricks?

GRANT (*nonchalantly*): No, I've been laying cold corpses. Forty in a day! The chaplain needed a helping hand. We wrapped them all in sailcloth and laid them in rows, based on ascending rank. Tomorrow will be a perfect day for a mass burial – cold and clear.

FLORENCE: How can you predict such things?

GRANT (*gestures upward*): I look at the stars. Their clarity tells a great deal about the atmospheric fluctuations.

Florence sighs and leans into Grant, her head almost touching his shoulder.

FLORENCE: Thank you.

GRANT: For the lesson in meteorology?

FLORENCE: No, for not ruining a perfectly scientific moment with poetic drivel. You had an opportunity to spout something nauseating about (*deliberates for a second*) cosmos, and infinity – yet you withstood the temptation. For that I am grateful.

7

GRANT: I assure you such thoughts did not even cross my mind. In turn, I am grateful for not having a mass burial in rainy weather with water destroying freshly dug graves. I looked up, and the stars told me what I wanted to know.

They look at each other.

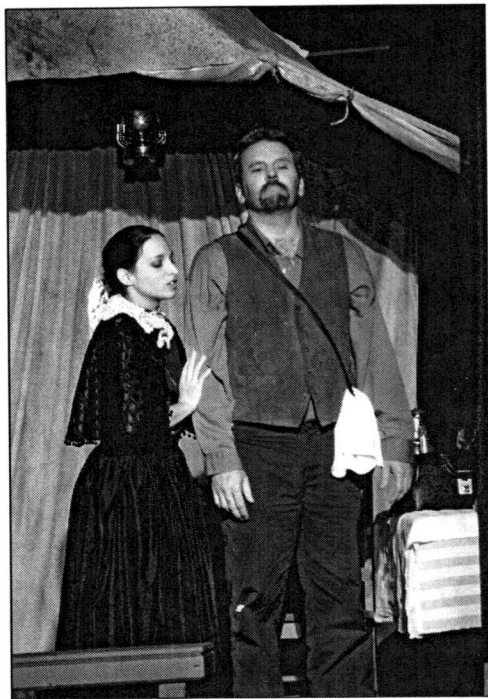

FLORENCE (*With a mixture of amusement and embarrassment*): Did you know I was once courted by a poet? Richard Milnes, Baron Houghton.

GRANT (*impressed*): A baron?

FLORENCE: A sentimental dolt! And a clumsy liar too. How he swore he wouldn't interfere with my practice! He even donated a sum to the hospital. Yet I knew it was only to cajole me into marriage. Had he attained his goal, all his false interest in my work would dissipate. (*Wags her hand*) Ah, he's married now. (*Boastfully and flirtatiously*) That does not prevent him from writing to me on occasion.

GRANT (*with mock pity*): Ah, poor Richard!

FLORENCE (*indignantly*): Poor Florence! Those self-proclaimed connoisseurs of the female soul know nothing about the female body. The man kissed as if he were afraid of poisoning me. Is it such a crime on my part to desire a skillful, well-executed kiss that isn't followed by a poetic couplet? (*Categorically, crossing her arms*)

GRANT (*fist in the air*): I endorse your righteous indignation!

8

FLORENCE (*relieved and sincerely appreciative*): I knew you would.

GRANT: Abstinence is next to idleness. Together, they cause insomnia and fits of hysteria. Like men, women need physical work and physical pleasure.

FLORENCE (*throws her arms up*): Amen! I attempted to communicate those simple medical facts to my dear Mama, and she howled that she had never heard such obscenities from a lady.

GRANT (*echoes*): From a lady...

FLORENCE: According to Mama, the sole purpose of my endeavors was to humiliate the family. In her eyes it was all a spectacle, a prolonged adolescent rebellion. A spoiled privileged girl experimenting with charity, poking beggars and orphans, dirtying her hands only to enrage her mother. What can be said in my defense? That's the kind of unfeeling ogress I am. (*With humorous self-deprecation*) I have a turnip in place of a heart.

GRANT (*pensively*): A turnip in place of a heart... Is that your expression?

FLORENCE: No, that's what Richard stated in his last letter to me. He does not recover from rejection quickly. (*Nostalgically*) And then there was Sidney Herbert, a divine man in every way – but married.

GRANT: You saw that as an obstacle?

FLORENCE: I didn't – but he did. Amusingly, years ago, when Sidney was free, he had an affair with a married woman. But now he won't betray his own wife, (*with a sense of superiority*) even though she disappoints him, and temptation is so near. Believe it or not, it was his initiative to send me to Crimea. He thought it would be prudent to put some distance between us. His wife was relieved, I'm certain. Sidney had joked about marrying me, should he suddenly become widowed. It's a hellishly awkward situation, and there will be no relief as long as all three of us are alive. One of us must die, or...

GRANT: Or you could find yourself a new lover. That would be a far more peaceful and pleasant solution.

FLORENCE: I wish it were so easy. I was impossible to impress in the past, but after meeting Sidney... How should I put it in scientific terms? Having tasted of morphine, how can one return to opium? I just know I shall die alone, a victim of my own fantastic standards. (*Rubs her eyes, embarrassed by her moment of weakness*) Forgive me, Dr. Grant. It is awfully rude of me to burden you with my complaints. You need not hear any of this.

GRANT: I'm accustomed to hearing all sorts of confessions from my patients. They mistake me for the chaplain. One of the lads from Donegal caught me by the waistcoat and sang a mournful ditty from his native village – in Gaelic. But, Miss Nightingale... I wish I could lift your spirits. (*Lifts finger up*) I know! I have a perfect book for you.

Florence shakes up and moves closer to Grant.

FLORENCE: Oh, what's the title?

GRANT: "England on Her Deathbed."

FLORENCE: And the author?

GRANT (*bows*): Yours truly.

FLORENCE: I am not astonished one bit. (*Pompously*) Where can I procure this masterpiece?

GRANT: Oh, it hasn't been completed it. I'll be sure to give you the final version before sending it to the printer. Imagine decades of medical journals, depicting everything from epidemics to opium addiction. There you'll find the most peculiar deaths of various English citizens, including my own children.

FLORENCE (*frowns incredulously*): You had children?

GRANT: Not by blood. It's long story... Those two entered my life after I had vowed not to pursue conventional fatherhood.

10

FLORENCE (*impatiently*): How they entered your life is immaterial to me. I only care to know how they departed. What was it: cholera, diphtheria?

GRANT: I fear you'll have to wait until the book is finished. The suspense will give you a reason to continue our friendly dialogue. I trade my knowledge for your company.

FLORENCE (*indignantly*): That is unpardonable cruelty, taunting me in this manner!

GRANT: Come now. I promised you will be the first one to read it. Until then, you'll have to muster all your patience.

FLORENCE (*defiantly*): In that case prepare to hear more unsavory confessions from me. By the end of this campaign you will be so satiated with my company that you will shove your unfinished manuscript into my hands just to be rid of me. Let's see whose patience runs out first.

GRANT: I accept the challenge.

Florence and Grant look at each other for a few seconds and then burst out laughing; Grant's laughter turns into cough. Florence's face assumes a more serious expression.

FLORENCE: Something must be done about this beastly growl.

GRANT (*dismissively*): Ah, it's nothing...

FLORENCE: That chamomile extract I gave you? Drink it. I spotted that flask on your night stand. It wasn't even opened. And fetch another pillow for your upper back. It will help you breathe. And open the window, even though it's cold.

Enter Bennett, chin lifted.

BENNETT: It pains me to interrupt your intellectual tryst, (*To Florence*) but Miss Nightingale, you better attend to Private Martin. Soon he will be waving his stump and screaming out your name.

Florence examines Martin one last time.

GRANT: You better rest. I'll send for someone to watch the patients.

FLORENCE (*to Grant*): Now, remember my instructions. This is no joking matter. You're one cough away from pneumonia.

Florence throws one more glance at Grant and leaves. Bennett tilts his head disdainfully behind Florence's back.

BENNETT: There she goes: the Joan of Arc of English medicine!

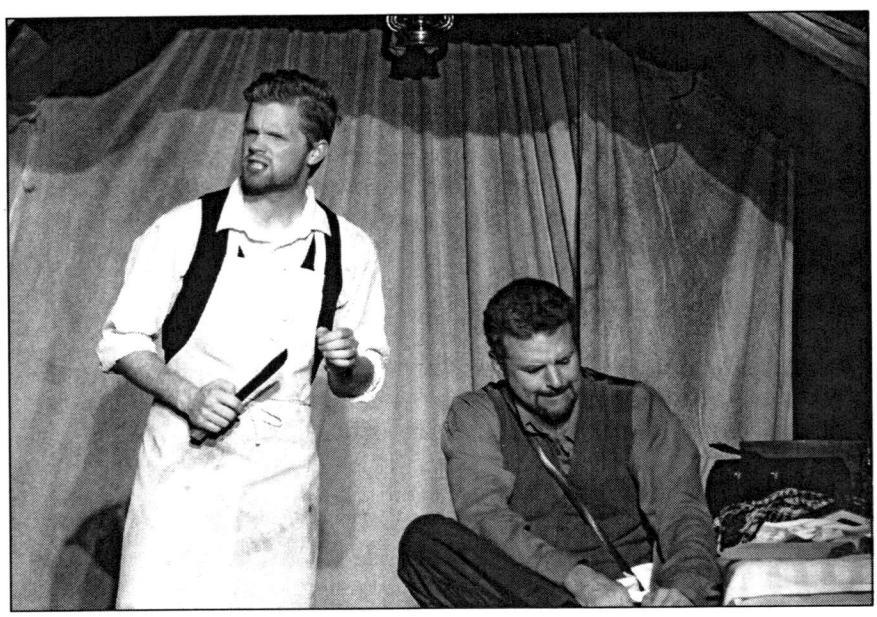

GRANT (*sternly*): Mr. Bennett, I wish you would show more courtesy to your female colleagues.

BENNETT: You mean – my female subordinates? As far as I recall, surgeons still rank somewhat above nurses, (*tone changes from sarcastic to hostile*) who in turn rank only somewhat above common whores.

GRANT: Well, since you raised the question of hierarchy, I am forced to remind you that I am still your superior. But, hierarchy aside, I implore you, as a fellow-gentleman--

12

BENNETT: You still classify yourself a gentleman? Thomas Grant, the Famished Bear!

GRANT: Bravo! I see you've done your detective work.

BENNETT: I know why you lost your medical license: you nearly killed a young patient, Lord Middleton's nephew. So you spent the last two decades in Southwark trading opium, sleeping between two circus girls and sheltering criminals in your home.

GRANT (*nods*): Yes, very well-researched. Some of those events took place before you were even born. Your interest in ancient history is commendable.

Bennett draws back and shakes his head incredulously.

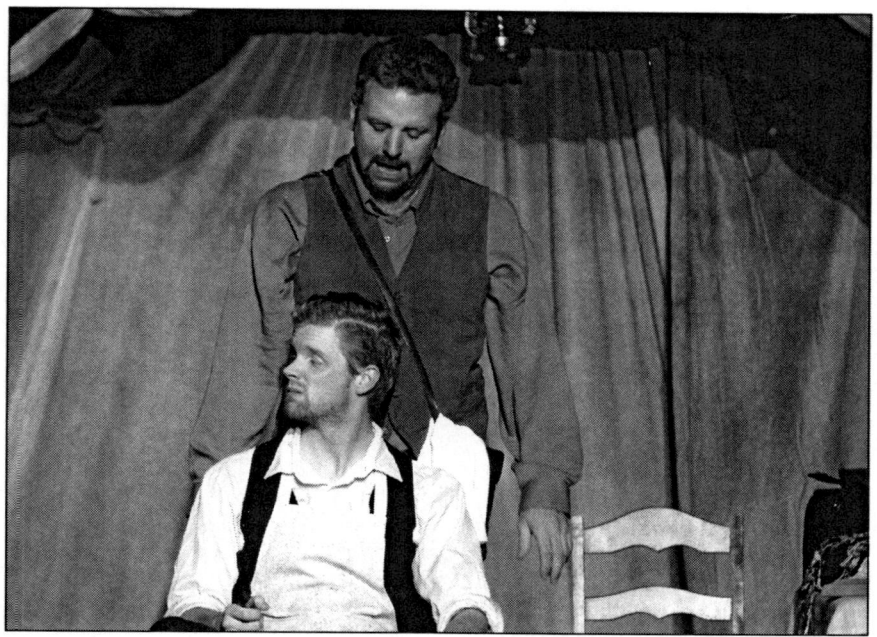

BENNETT: What? You have nothing to say in your defense? For God's sake, have you no instinct for self-preservation?

GRANT: If I had any such instinct left, would I have sailed to the Crimea?

BENNETT (*points finger triumphantly*): Oh, I see where this is leading! It's all perfectly logical. After indulging in every perversion under the sun, the Famished Bear resorts to a life of asceticism. He has no instincts! (*Opens his arms and lifts them*) He has transcended them!

GRANT: Can't you admit being envious of my colorful and adventurous past? (*Patronizingly*) Don't despair, my young friend. You too will have a reputation some day. I need not defend myself before anyone. It may disappoint you, but all my misdemeanors are common knowledge. I have no secrets. I have no shame. However, I still have an obligation to my patients, which brings me to the subject of Private Martin, whose hand you amputated earlier. I had specifically instructed you to remove the index finger above the joint. How do you explain your (*pause*)... improvisation?

BENNETT: The hand was gangrenous! Another day - and we'd have to amputate up to the elbow. Two days – up to the shoulder. Three days – and he'd be dead.

GRANT: Mr. Bennett, your youthful imagination paints all sorts of Shakespearean catastrophes. I examined the patient this morning. The hand was perfectly salvageable. You crippled a man for no reason. It was my decision to make – not yours.

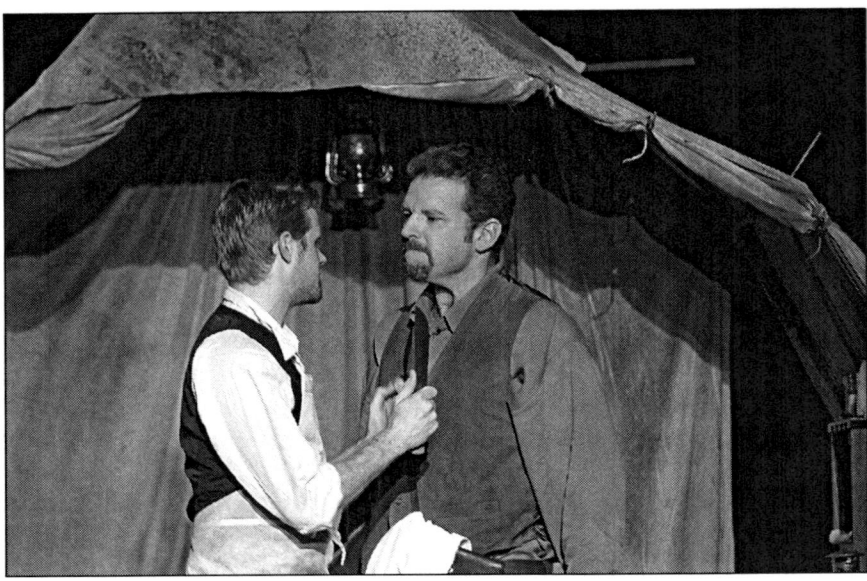

BENNETT: You are not fit to make such decisions! And I shall make sure that everyone knows it. You'll go back to trading opium and helping slum whores get rid of their unwanted offspring.

GRANT (*rubs his chin defiantly*): I've been alive for half a century. Over the course of that time, many wars have been waged against me. Yet I'm still alive, which cannot be said for my adversaries. It is God's will that I should remain in this world and in this profession. You may want to consider that, Mr. Bennett, before your next attempt to remove me from your path.

They both exit. Lights fade.

Scene 3

Lights up; early morning. Inside the surgical tent, Private Martin rises from his bed, his arm in a sling, the stump of his amputated hand wrapped in a bloodied cloth. He wavers, still under the effects of the chloroform anesthesia. Rebecca enters, carrying clean linens. She gasps, startled.

REBECCA: Mr. Martin, what are you doing out of bed?

MARTIN: I grew bored starin' upward. I see a deep shadow movin' 'cross the ceilin'. I see hell's gate openin' up to suck me in. I'm not ready to go yet. The idiot chaplain hasn't stopped by to absolve me.

REBECCA: You shouldn't be walking. You've lost too much blood.

MARTIN: When I'm on me feet, I don't think 'bout the missin' hand. And then I try to light a cigar... And I remember I've no tobacco. Someone emptied me pockets.

REBECCA: I regret your loss, Mr. Martin.

MARTIN: The tobacco?

REBECCA (*annoyed by his joke*): No, your hand.

MARTIN (*examines his stump*): This is no great loss, not fer England. Even b'fore this happened I was useless. Me dead Ma will testify to that. Now, with only one hand left, I'm half the thief.

17

(*Laughs like a madman, causing Rebecca to draw back*) Sweet Rebecca, don't flee. You needn't fear me.

REBECCA: I don't fear you. I fear *for* you. The sedatives make you rant.

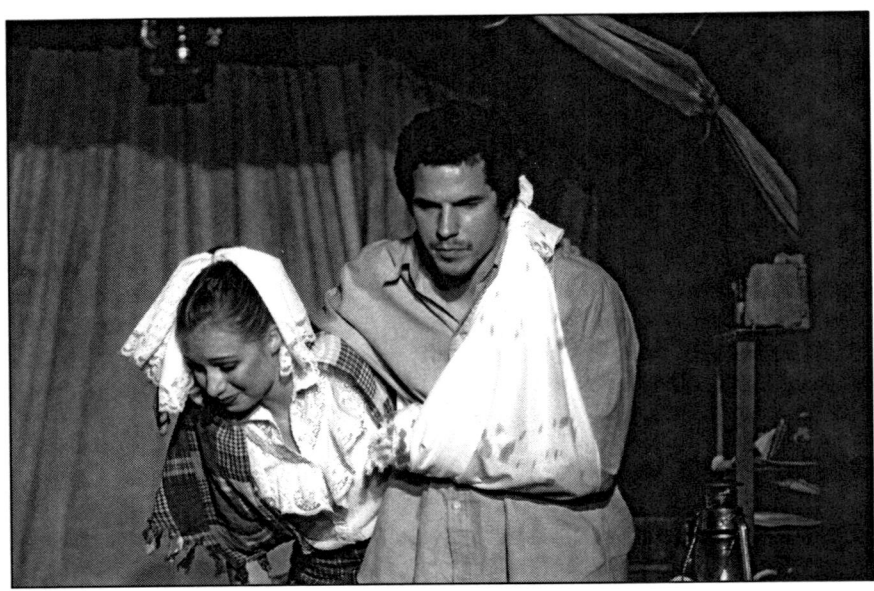

MARTIN: Those drugs didn't do a bloody thin' save blur me eyesight. I recall the lantern danglin' 'bove me head, fadin' out and blazin' up again. I recall seein' yer face, green and twisted, and hearin' yer scream, that very scream I m'self was denied, as I lay there, strapped to the table, me hand on the choppin' board and a block of wood 'tween me teeth. 'Twas yer first time, eh?

REBECCA (*lowers her eyes with embarrassment*): And last. Mr. Bennett says I'm not to enter the surgical tent again.

MARTIN: That butcher exiled you? Surely, he wants to fill the tent wi' his own kind. Lucky is 'e that I'm crippled. Wouldn't I love to take 'im by the throat... Put me both thumbs right there (*points to the hollow under his Adam's apple*). There's many a man I'd like to strangle, not just the surgeon. All of 'em... Don't yer know, that clown, Lord Card'gan, is drinkin' 'himself stupid on 'is yacht. Not a hair on 'is bloody head was harmed. But the man trembles b'fore

18

Lord Lucan, and Lucan trembles b'fore Lord Raglan. In short, we've got a chain of tremblin' cowards, murderers they be!

REBECCA: Be careful, Mr. Martin, saying such things...

MARTIN: But yer see, love, I'm not the only one sayin' such thins. Yer ought to hear the lads in the tent. If I be shot for speakin' my mind, they may as well shoot the entire Light Brigade – well, whatev'r is left of it... There's a mut'ny brewin'. Unluck'ly, I won't partake in it. I'm sailn' home soon. 'Tis costly to feed a useless cripple. Every breadcrumb is accounted for, yer know. They promise me twenty pounds fer the damages. P'haps I'll change me trade. I'll buy a hook for me stump and a parrot for me shoulder and frighten 'em children by the docks. I already know plenty of robber songs. Now I'll learn a few pirate songs. (*With mock gallantry*) Until then, Rebecca, I shall remain your most devoted vassal.

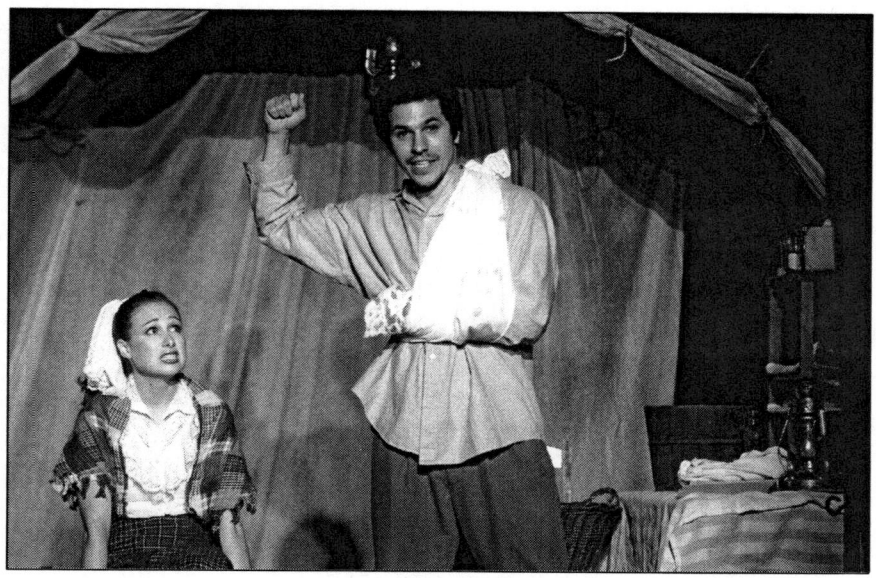

Martin grabs Rebecca's hand and brings it to his lips. Then he loses his balance and falls into her lap. Rebecca gasps with a mixture of terror and disgust.

19

REBECCA: Mr. Martin, you're bleeding! Your wound... (*Grabs her head in bewilderment*) What am I to do? (*Screams frantically*) Miss Nightingale! Someone, come, help me!

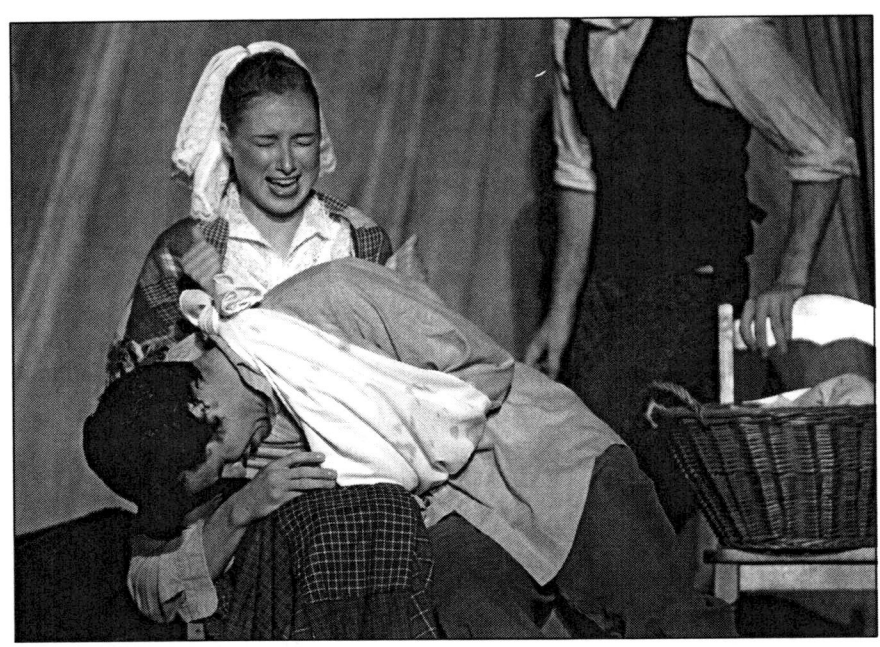

Bennett enters, surveys the scene for a few seconds, grabs Martin by the scruff of his neck and pulls him up roughly from Rebecca's lap.

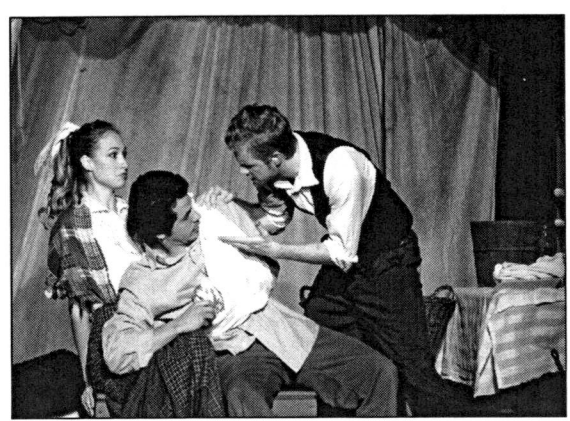

BENNETT: Do you want gangrene to spread, ah? One amputation wasn't enough for you? Perhaps, you want me to repeat the procedure?

MARTIN (*defiantly, into Bennett's face*): Oh, wouldn't yer love that... choppin' up yer victims inch by inch.

BENNETT: If you don't stop ranting, I'll cut off your tongue too.

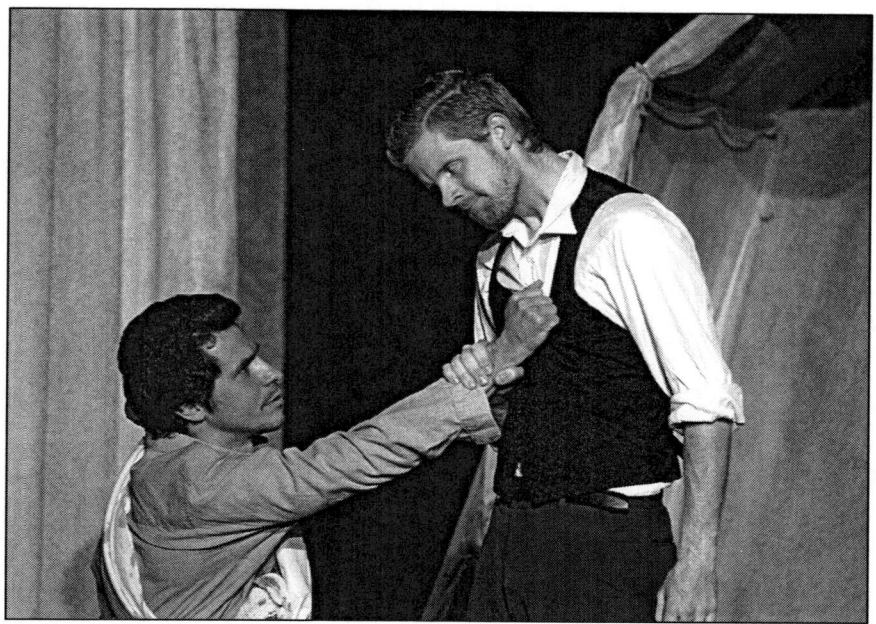

Bennett glares at Rebecca, shakes Martin one more time and drags him back to bed and exits. Rebecca goes to check on Martin. Lights fade.

Scene 4

A stateroom on Lord Cardigan's yacht. Cardigan is sitting in his arm chair, clutching a bottle of brandy. He hears the door creak and twitches. Enter Grant his body posture communicating great unease and reluctance. Cardigan puts the brandy bottle behind the chair, stands up and opens his arms with extravagant familiarity.

CARDINGAN: Ah, Ted!

GRANT (*coldly*): Tom.

CARDIGAN (*slowly, as if addressing an idiot*): No, my name is Jim.

Grant struggles to maintain dignity and diplomacy, then responds, mimicking Cardigan's condescending tone.

GRANT: I am aware of that – your Lordship. (*Taps his chest*) I am Tom... Thomas Henry Grant, doctor of medicine and philosophy. (*Straightens out*) Reporting for duty – Your Lordship...

CARDIGAN: Well, Thomas Henry Grant, do you know why you were summoned here?

GRANT: I dare not fathom, Your Lordship.

Cardigan paces around his stateroom; Grant remains standing.

CARDIGAN: So tell me: how do you like your occupation?

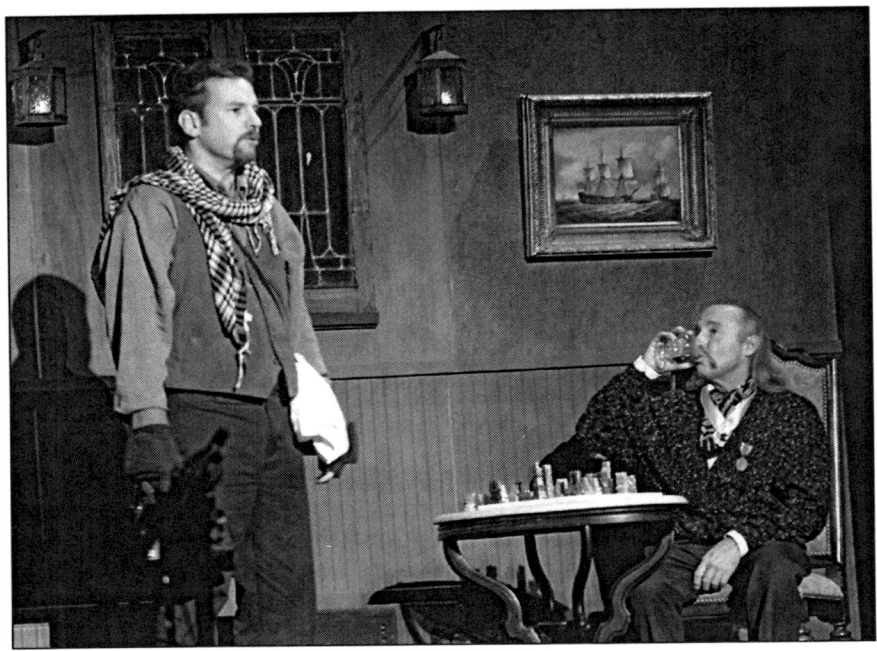

GRANT (*reluctantly*): I am honored to serve my country.

CARDIGAN (*rolls his eyes*): Bah! I would've expected a more original answer from you. (*Mocking pompously*) "Honored to serve my country..." At any rate, your service won't continue much longer.

GRANT: Why is that, Your Lordship?

CARDIGAN: I've been conversing with Mr. Bennett.

GRANT: Oh...

CARDIGAN: He was kind enough to inform me about your past practices.

GRANT (*rubs the back of his head*): What exactly has he told you?

CARDIGAN (*flicks his wrist casually*): Only good things - your fondness for Bohemian women, your selective adherence to the law, your intimate knowledge of narcotics. Clearly, a man like you does not belong in a military hospital.

24

GRANT: It grieves me infinitely to hear that, Your Lordship. If only I could persuade you to rethink your decision...

CARDIGAN: Let me finish. A man like you should not squander his time, talent and knowledge on the sort of tasks you've been performing for the past month. He should serve his country on a higher level.

GRANT (*fearfully*): Exactly, how high?

CARDIGAN (*in a businesslike manner*): How much do you know about sedatives?

GRANT (*nods*): Enough.

CARDIGAN (*mysteriously, all-knowingly*): I have a family member in dire need of sedation. (*Dragging out vowels*) Deep sedation...

GRANT (*frowns, perplexed*): I am afraid, I do not understand...

CARDIGAN (*irritated*): You know perfectly well of whom I speak! Lord Lucan, my brother-in-law! The fault is all his, you know.

GRANT: What fault?

CARDIGAN: The damn charge of the Light Brigade, naturally! My dear brother-in-law botched the campaign. (*Vindictively*) It is his choleric temper and incompetent leadership that cost us so many soldiers. He sent us in the wrong direction. Of course, he'll attempt to put all blame on me, coward that he is. He's always hated me. Lord Raglan has demanded a private audience with him. It won't astonish me if poor old George is court-martialed.

GRANT: So, how does my pharmaceutical expertise fit into your vengeance plan? Am I expected to poison Lord Lucan?

CARDIGAN: Of course not! I want him alive, to watch him reap his shame in full. I want him debilitated, unable to lead another Englishman to his death. (*Lifts his index finger, having gotten a brilliant idea*) Better yet! Instead of a sedative, give him a hallucinogenic. Turn him into a raving lunatic. (*Rubs his hands in evil*

25

delight, then throws his arm around Grant's neck, hanging on him) Yes, yes... Humiliate him before his subordinates and superiors, his mistresses and his bastard offspring. I know where he stores his wine bottles.

GRANT (*moves away from Cardigan*): Your Lordship, I do not believe that you are in the condition to plan such intricate retaliation. Perhaps, we could continue our audience at a better time, when your mind is a bit more lucid.

CARDIGAN: You think I am drunk? I'm perfectly sober! You haven't seen me drunk, my friend. I only took a few sips of brandy to warm up. Would you like some? Perhaps, that will place us on the same altitude. In no time, you shall be thinking and behaving like Cardigan!

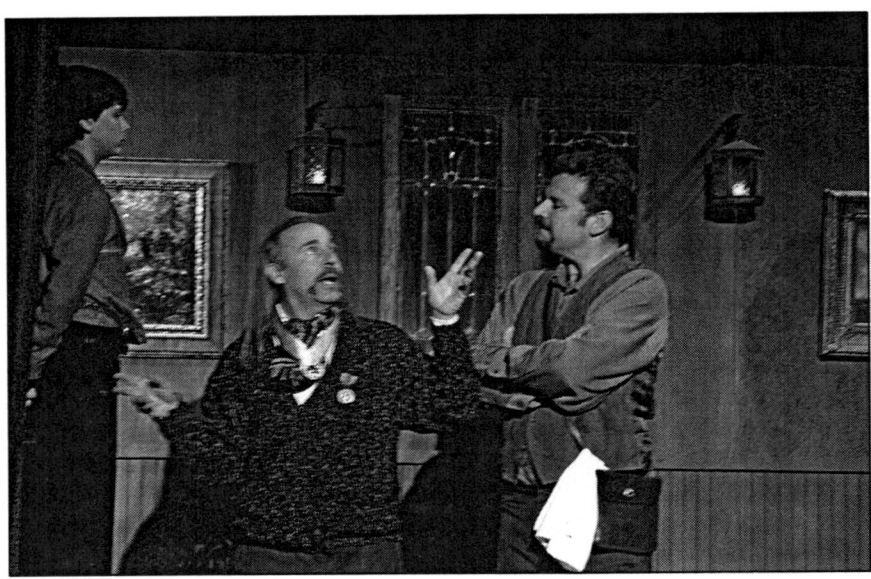

GRANT (*mumbles*): Oh, joy...

Cardigan grabs his bottle, his hands still trembling, pours a drink for Grant.

CARDIGAN: Do you see, Tom? I pour my own brandy with my own hands for you. Tell me, Tom. When you were in Southwark, did you think you would ever find yourself on the most splendid yacht, in the presence of England's greatest general? I'm almost envious of you. To rise so high in such a short segment of time.

Lucan comes in. Cardigan twitches, visibly disturbed.

CARDIGAN: What are you doing on my yacht, George?

LUCAN: I was about to ask you the same question, James? How long do you think you could hide from the world?

CARDIGAN: I am not hiding. I am recovering.

LUCAN: I see... (*Points at Grant disdainfully*): What is this?

CARDIGAN: This? This is my new chum, Tom Grant.

Cardigan pushes Grant forward and hides behind him.

LUCAN (*cheerfully*): Ah, the pioneer of human vivisection! Cambridge is famous for producing mad scientists.

GRANT (*coughs*): Lord Lucan, forgive my intrusion, but I would like to contest those allegations. I have never cut a living being without an explicit consent.

LUCAN (*dismissively*): Good doctor, your wild experiments are none of my concern. I have more important issues to ponder than a few dismembered orphans. (*To Cardigan, menacingly*) James, you know well that you and I have a lengthy discussion ahead of us. I'd like the pleasure of your brotherly company for the next four or five hours. So get rid of the evil genius.

CARDIGAN: The evil genius is treating my injuries.

Cardigan grabs his shoulder and makes a grimace of pain.

LUCAN: Ah, those the injuries you sustained while riding back from the front lines, as the men in your command rode to their deaths? You can show those injuries to Lord Raglan during our audience tomorrow. Anything to prove your courage and determination!

27

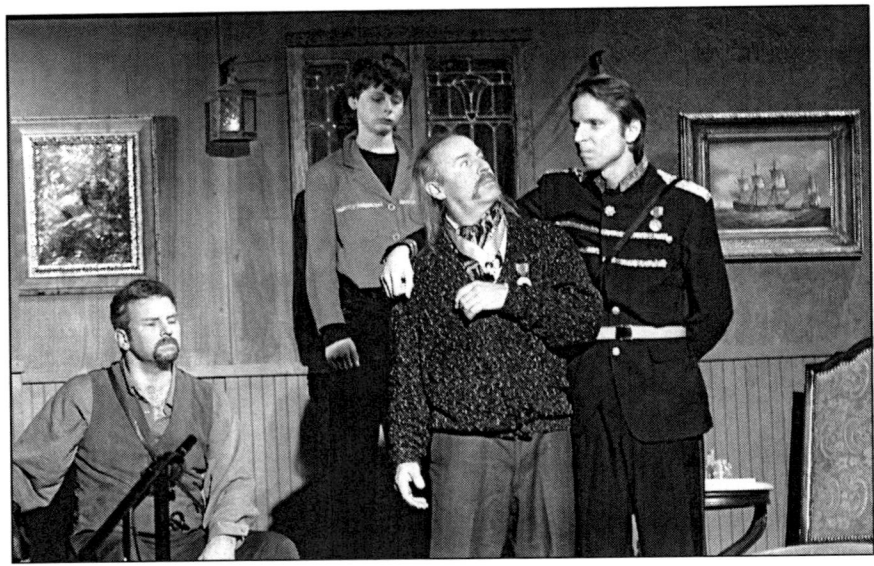

CARDIGAN: My presence was not requested. It is not my custom to go where I am not invited. I have no doubt that you will relate your version of the story coherently.

LUCAN (*with mock affection*): But I want you to be by my side, Jimmy. You are my right hand, the one that doesn't always follow the commands of the brain. I've grown to find your stupidity endearing. It adds excitement to the dull military routine. I never quite know what my darling Jim will pull on the battlefield. This mystery is what keeps me in the saddle. And at this moment I am relying on your brotherly love to do what is asked of you. Do not make me employ my status as your superior.

CARDIGAN: But George, if we stand side by side, the thin ice beneath our feet will surely crack.

LUCAN: The ice has already cracked, my dear. I'm already up to my chin in water. And as I go under, it would

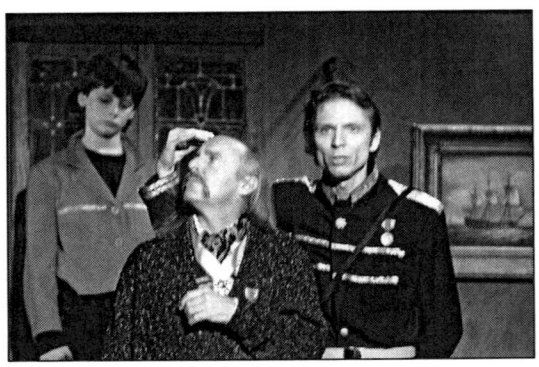

28

be comforting to know that you too are drowning, not far from me.

Grant, desperately trying to bring comic relief, points at the revolver sticking out from under Lucan's belt.

GRANT: Is that a Model Adams? Excellent choice! You know, my son used to extract those guns from the factory in London. He's dead now. But when he was alive, he was quite a metal scavenger. You should've seen the oddities he brought home from the streets.

Cardigan laughs hysterically in support of Grant's jokes and hides behind his back. Lucan moves in menacingly.

LUCAN (*to Cardigan*): You think this haggard mass of bones and chest hair can protect you? Quite a bodyguard you've found! A sickly bear with red eyes... Will he dare to raise his claw in your defense, against me? This is why you invited him here, didn't you? So you wouldn't have to be alone, with me...

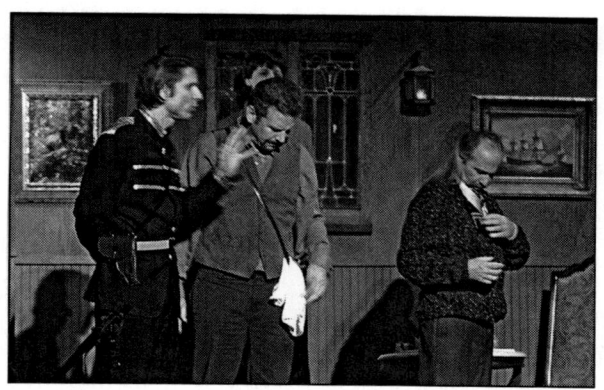

Lucan leaps forward, reaches behind Grant's back, pulls Cardigan by the front of his shirt and knocks him down with one punch to the jaw. Cardigan reaches his hand out towards Grant, begging for protection, but Lucan steps on his hand. Grant remains standing still; his breathing quickens.

LUCAN (*to Grant*): Watch this, good doctor. After all, what else can you do? Here's an intimate moment in English history, something for you to discuss in the surgical tent with your butcher colleagues.

29

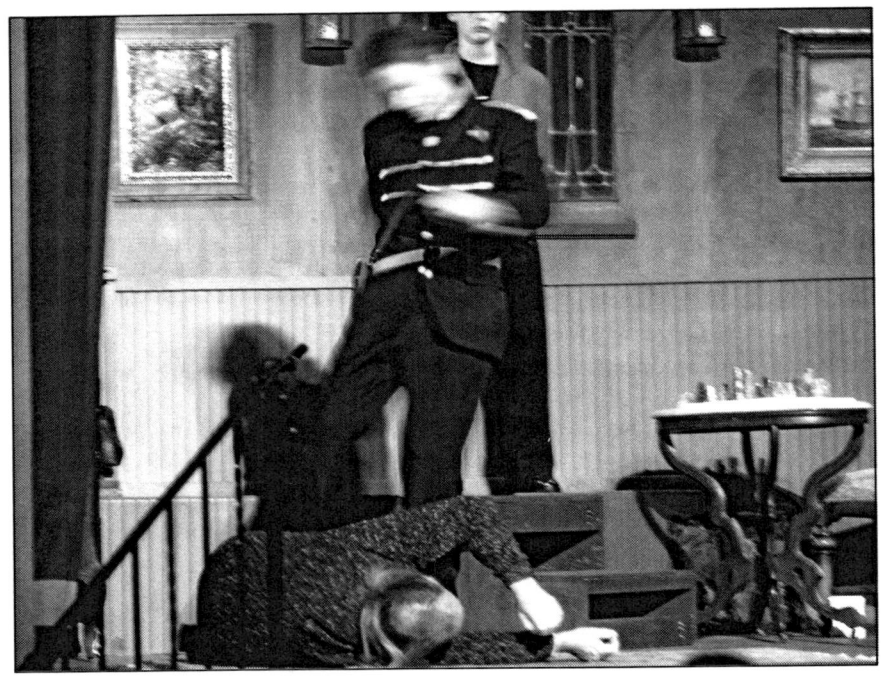

Lucan kicks Cardigan a few times and then backs off abruptly.

LUCAN: There's no sport battering a drunk. Good doctor, do your duty. My brother-in-law will need a few cold compresses. Thus he won't need to fake his injuries for the audience tomorrow. His pain will look more authentic.

Lucan turns around and leaves, fetching the half-empty bottle of brandy on his way out. Cardigan twitches on the floor, wincing in pain. Grant comes to his senses, shakes up and helps Cardigan to his chair.

CARDIGAN: Now you see that he is perfectly insane.

GRANT: All I see is that you and your brother-in-law have much to sort out.

Cardigan gestures in the direction in which Lucan had left moments ago.

30

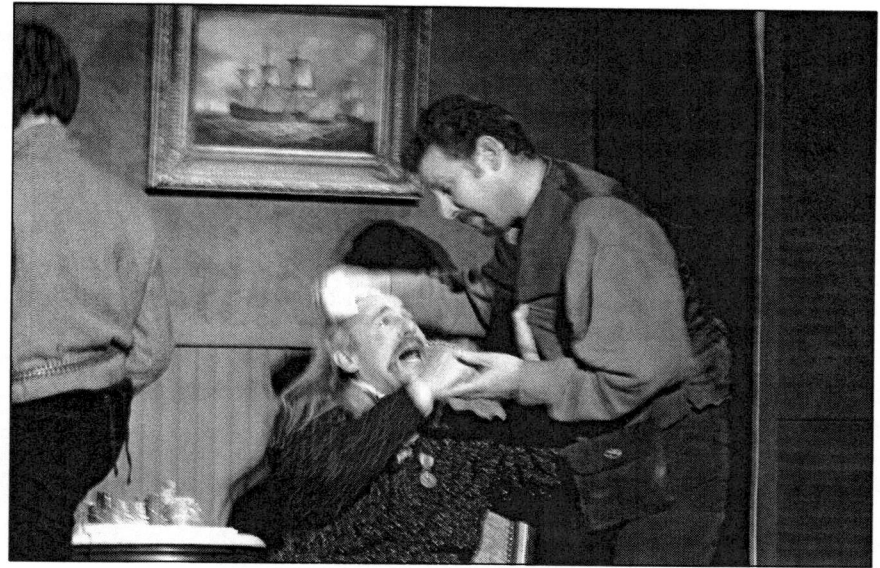

CARDIGAN: Tom, I can't reason with the man. He won't respond to logic. But he will respond to your concoction. It is our only hope.

Grant straightens out abruptly and backs away from Cardigan.

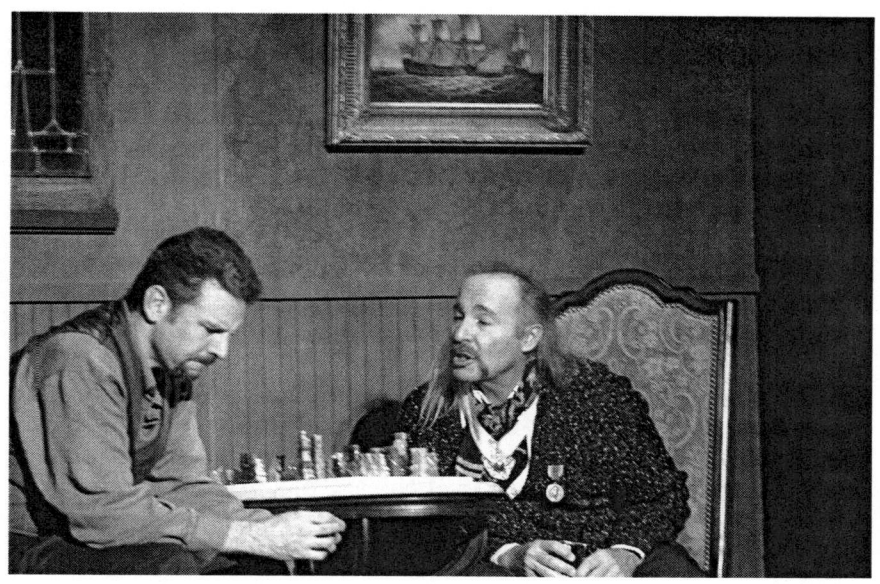

GRANT (*self-deprecatingly*): On another thought, I must confess that my knowledge of the apothecary field has been over-praised. I do not know that much about sedatives after all. Perhaps, you should recruit someone more experienced. It sounds like an awfully important mission, and I would hate to botch it.

CARDIGAN: Tom, you are a pitiable liar!

GRANT (*sighs, resuming a sincere tone*): This is precisely why I am a doctor and not a politician. (*Pause*) Honestly, Your Lordship, I should not partake in this plot.

CARDIGAN: Leave the plotting to me. Your duty is to mix the potion.

GRANT: My Lord, you put me in a most unenviable position.

CARDIGAN: But then, whose position is enviable, do tell? You know any men who sleep well at night?

GRANT: The chaplain! He dumps the corpses in a mass grave, blurts out a prayer and snores away the night. A job well-done...

CARDIGAN: I mean men of importance, men whose names are mentioned in history tomes. Tom, as much as I detest resorting to such bluntness, you have no choice. You aren't leaving my yacht pretending that his conversation had not taken place.

GRANT (*sternly and defiantly*): My Lord, as much as I detest resorting to such bluntness, you have no power over me. This ragged old puppet's strings have been cut long ago. I do not fear for my own life. As for my loved ones, they are all dead.

CARDIGAN (*raises his index finger*): That is not entirely true. Mr. Bennett told me that you've been growing quite chummy with a certain nurse.

GRANT: You mean, Florence Nightingale? She means nothing to me. A conceited spinster... I am not saying that she is entirely useless. A pair of hands... But there's nothing about her to capture my fancy. I do not pursue women over the age of thirty.

CARDIGAN (*shakes his head reproachfully*): Ah, Tom... One day, I'll teach you to lie with a straight face. Until then, don't make any attempts. You are in love with Florence Nightingale! And why wouldn't you be? She is an exceptional woman. And you (*points at Grant*) are an exceptional man.

GRANT: I can't compete with Sidney Herbert.

CARDIGAN: And Florence can't compete with Sidney Herbert's wife. It's hopeless. I'm privy to the situation. Sidney is another close chum of mine. He shall never divorce or betray Elizabeth. For that I can vouch. In the meantime, our saintly Florence, the Lady with the Lamp, has nothing left to do except pray secretly for her rival's death and grow mad little by little. Ah, the demon voices in her weary little head... It would be a crime to leave her in such a perilous state. She needs somebody seasoned, witty and commanding to distract her from her unhealthy fantasies – someone like you.

GRANT (*with embarrassment*): Why, Lord Cardigan, I don't think I've received so many compliments from another man in my entire life.

CARDIGAN (*mysteriously*): But wait: I have more than mere compliments to offer.

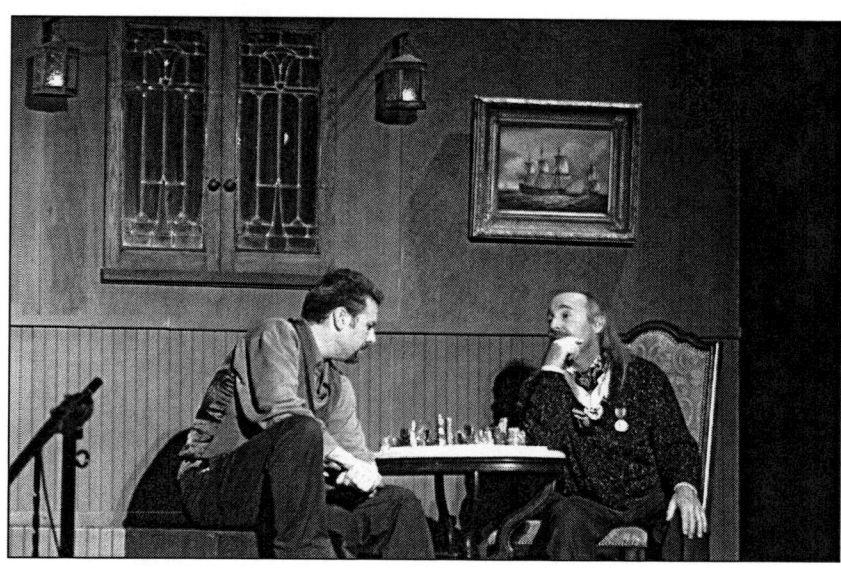

33

GRANT (*with growing unrest*): What exactly did you have in mind, my lord?

CARDIGAN: How about ten thousand pounds as a modest appetizer? The sum may seem fantastic to you now, as you haven't adopted my habits yet. But you shall learn to burn through money with breathtaking elegance. And if you do not care for money, I shall find other ways to compensate you. Imagine having a splendid laboratory in Westminster, and all the leisure and comfort in the world for your intellectual endeavors. Imagine being surrounded by dazzling minds. You will not need to seek them – they shall seek you. A few words from me - and all the young medical prodigies of England shall flock to you. And Florence shall be by your side all the while. I shall advocate for that stubborn girl. You two can become the golden couple of English medicine. Now tell me that all this is not worth a small flask of potion?

Grant suddenly wavers, clutches his chest with one hand and with another hand leans on the back of Cardigan's armchair.

GRANT (*faintly*): Forgive me, your Lordship... I have been unwell for a few days. There's an infectious cough in the hospital corps. If you don't believe me...

CARDIGAN: No, this time I believe you. Dear friend, you must preserve your strength. We have much work ahead of us.

Cardigan hastily vacates the armchair and helps Grant sit down.

Scene 5

Outside a surgical tent, Private Martin is on the bench, clutching the stump of his hand, rocking back and forth and moaning, his eyes wild. Florence holds him by the shoulders from behind, trying to console him.

MARTIN (*rants wildly*): It burns... Me hand burns! From the elbow to... where the fingertips once were. The hand's gone, but the pain stays.

FLORENCE: Hapless boy...

MARTIN: I asked 'im fer drugs, I begged 'im. But he'd give me none!

FLORENCE: Who?

MARTIN: The bloody surgeon... I hate 'im! I could kill 'im, I swear. The bastard, he passes by, grinnin', mockin' me...

Florence draws a small flask from her bag and holds it to Martin's lips.

FLORENCE: Here's some valerian root. It can't hurt. Drink up.

Martin takes a few sips and collapses, breathing heavily, as Florence cradles him like a child and strokes his hair. After a few seconds Martin calms down.

MARTIN: Talk to me. 'Bout anythin'. I only need to hear yer voice.

35

FLORENCE (*with forced optimism*): Just think: you'll be sent home soon. But first you'll receive your pay. Spend your money wisely. Consult your mother.

MARTIN: She died whilst I was in pris'n.

FLORENCE: Ah, the whole world is a prison. Just because you aren't chained, it doesn't mean that you are free.

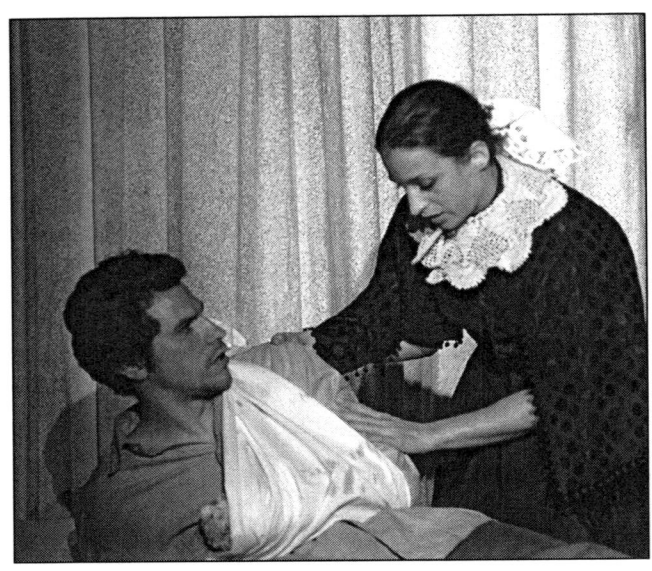

Martin notices a corner of an envelope peeking from the collar of Florence's blouse.

MARTIN: A letter, eh?

FLORENCE: From a dear old friend.

MARTIN: What's his name?

FLORENCE (*faintly, staring into space*): Sidney.

MARTIN: Does 'e have any good news?

FLORENCE: It's an old letter, filled with promises yet to be ful-filled. When I have a dismal day, I reread it.

36

MARTIN: 'Tis pity I'm unlettered.

FLORENCE: I'll teach you how to scribble your name. Your writing hand is unharmed. (*Squeezes his right hand*) There's no excuse for continuing to communicate in muffled grunts. I hope that your writing will be more articulate than your speech.

MARTIN: Where's Dr. Grant?

FLORENCE: He was sent back to England. I was informed earlier in the morning.

MARTIN: Why?

FLORENCE: I can only guess. Another friend leaving my side... I should've expected something of the sort. The moment I find a worthy conversation partner, someone who can construct elaborate phrases and use Latin terms, he is snatched from me.

MARTIN: And that's why yer day's dismal?

Martin's body grows limp. He starts falling asleep. Florence continues stroking his hair, talking to herself rather than to him.

FLORENCE: He better make himself known when this travesty is over. He better find me home in England, or I'll find him. He promised to give me his book. (*With female jealousy*) If I discover that he allowed another woman to read it first... So help him God! Oh, the sparkling dialogues we could've had. I can almost hear his cough behind my back. It's not unlike that lingering pain from a hand that's been severed.

Rebecca enters, wringing her hands nervously, mumbling indistinctly. Florence leaves Martin and pulls Rebecca aside.

FLORENCE (*arms crossed*): Miss Prior, you have exactly two minutes to spill your tribulations. I hope to God they are grave enough.

REBECCA: It's Mr. Bennett...

FLORENCE: Does he still scold you for that incident last week?

REBECCA: No, he hasn't spoken of that night. It's not his words. It's his glances. They leave me unsettled.

Florence looks down, covers her mouth, formulating an answer, inhales, nods, then looks up at Rebecca.

FLORENCE: Miss Prior, I can't fathom what I could have done to encourage this sort of familiarity between us, to position myself as your confidant. When you barged in I thought for an instant that there was an attack or a fire. You distract me from my patients only to inform me that Mr. Bennett's glances leave you unsettled? Why, do you think, he chose you of all women as his target?

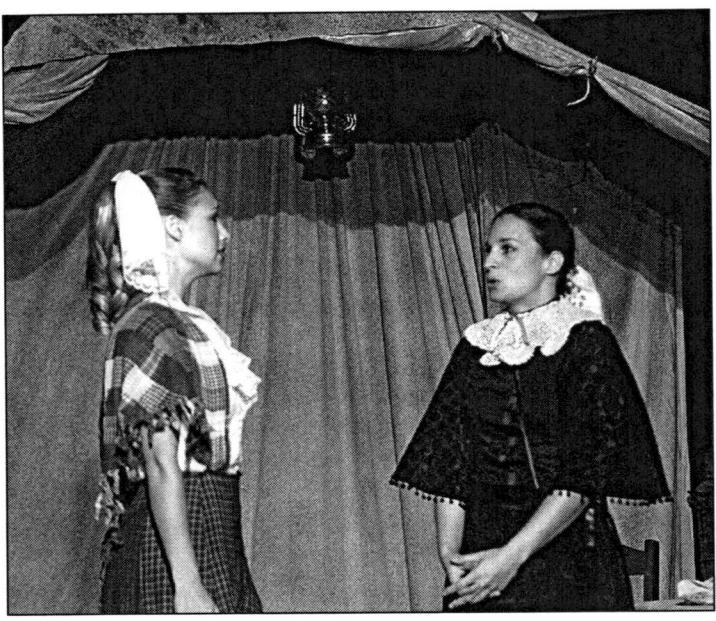

REBECCA (*Shrugs with contempt*): The rest of the nurses are nuns. Molly Fields and I are the only laywomen. Most of them are too bloody old, some well over thirty, and some (*shudders*) - over forty!

FLORENCE (*gasps in mock horror*): God forbid... What business they have being alive! The audacity, to last that long! You and Molly are like yellow-beaked fledglings among old hens. What a lonely life it must be for the two of you.

REBECCA: When Mr. Bennett stares at me, I simply can't work. My knees tremble, and my hands freeze.

FLORENCE: I think I know why your knees tremble, Miss Prior. There's a scientific explanation for it. (*Leans to Rebecca and sniffs the air*) Have you been drinking sterilizing solution?

REBECCA (*Raises her hands in defense*): I swear it's not my fault! It's Molly... She carries a whiskey flask.

FLORENCE (*Sarcastically*): And I suppose, Molly pried your jaws open and poured the content of the flask down your throat. And then she forcefully curled your hair (*tugs at Rebecca's hair*), and stuffed rolled-up gauze down your blouse (*tugs at the collar of Rebecca's blouse*), and smudged old rouge over your cheeks (*tilts Rebecca's chin*). What wayward, scandalous girl, that Molly is! Perhaps, I should have a private talk with her.

REBECCA (*Hastily*): Please, don't be cross with Molly. She mustn't worry in her condition.

FLORENCE: What condition? (*With disgust*) Oh, sweet mother of God... Not wasting any time, is she! Who's the lucky partner in crime?

REBECCA: She's not quite sure.

FLORENCE: Not quite sure? What a surprise! A fortunate baby, indeed! Some are born fatherless, but this one will have the entire Light Brigade for a father.

REBECCA: Molly was already in (*giggles awkwardly*) that way when she came here. For three days she vomited. We feared it was cholera... But it wasn't cholera. Imagine our relief. So Molly came to Dr. Grant in hopes that he would help her... put this mishap behind her. But he refused...

FLORENCE (*With growing disgust*): What possessed her to approach Dr. Grant with such a request?

REBECCA (*Matter-of-factly*): We've all heard about his past, his days in Southwark. There are all sorts of tales going around. But Dr. Grant swore that he had never rendered such services to women. He persuaded Molly to keep the baby and stop drinking. So she gave me her whiskey flask, and I gave her my shawl to hide her belly as it grows.

FLORENCE: Why, this is female solidarity at its finest! And then you wonder why Mr. Bennett stares at you. Look at yourself! You're a walking circus, drunk and painted while on duty! And then you run to me for protection! How do you expect me to protect you? I would have to dunk your head into a bucket of cold water first.

REBECCA (*on the brink of tears*): Miss Nightingale, I thought that you'd understand... Being a woman and all...

FLORENCE: I am not a woman - not in the sense that you and Molly are. Allow me to make myself clear. I am a sergeant in petticoats. Truth be told, I feel very little affection for women, weak and foolish ones in particular. Their lot does not concern me. If my work reflects well on them, if it raises their standing, it will merely be a fortunate coincidence. My mission is not to advocate for the females of the species. I've reaped no benefit from associating with them. I prefer the company of powerful men.

Rebecca nods feverishly, her attitude changing from imploring to aggressive.

REBECCA: I see now! You're envious of me, old maid that you are. Those big and mighty men of whom you speak – they won't bed you in a thousand years! That's right. They have no use for you. Wouldn't you love to trade places with me! Scrawny spinster... with a gray face and gray hairs...

Rebecca draws back, panting, terrified by her own outburst.

FLORENCE: Dear girl, if you carry on in this manner, you won't live to be an old maid. You will die a young hussy – if that is a more appealing fate.

Rebecca slouches and runs off. Martin stirs on his bed and raises himself on the elbow.

MARTIN: Was Rebecca here?

FLORENCE (*tersely*): Yes, she just left.

MARTIN: I knew I heard 'er voice, so near... Seen 'er shadow. Couldn't get me eyes to open.

FLORENCE: You were sleeping.

MARTIN (*resigned*): I s'ppose... But how heavenly 'twould be... Havin' her fer a mistress and you fer a mother... I'd be the jolliest one-armed thief in the whole of England.

His elbow gives in, and he falls back on the bench.

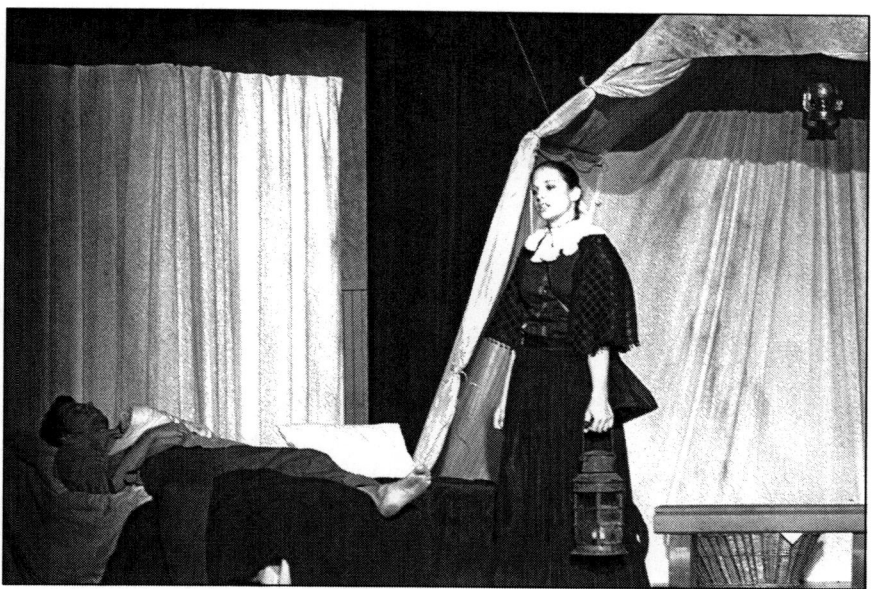

FLORENCE (*throws her arms in despair*): Why is it that every pickpocket under the sun considers me his mother? (*Stands over Martin*) Dear boy, if you were my son, you would've turned out quite differently, I assure you. For one, you would've developed a more discriminating taste in women.

MARTIN (*taken aback by her tone*): I don't understand...

FLORENCE: I don't expect you to understand. Perhaps, you and Rebecca would make a fine pair after all. You both have limited vocabularies and limited control over your impulses. Alas, I can't cure you of your origin. It is not in my power - or in my contract. I can only bandage your stump and pour some sedatives under your tongue. Let us not pamper our illusions. I am nobody's mother. I am but a frigid spinster. And you are an orphan, and a thief, and an invalid. And Rebecca is a hussy. What's even more tragic? We're all English citizens. We have allied with a Muslim nation against our fellow Christians. That alone can unsettle your stomach worse than cholera.

Florence exits, leaving Martin on the bed. Lights fade.

Scene 6

Lucan in his morning coat is smoking his cigar. Bennett is standing by his side, head bowed, hands clasped to his chest, exuding servility.

BENNETT: Thank you, my lord, for granting me this audience.

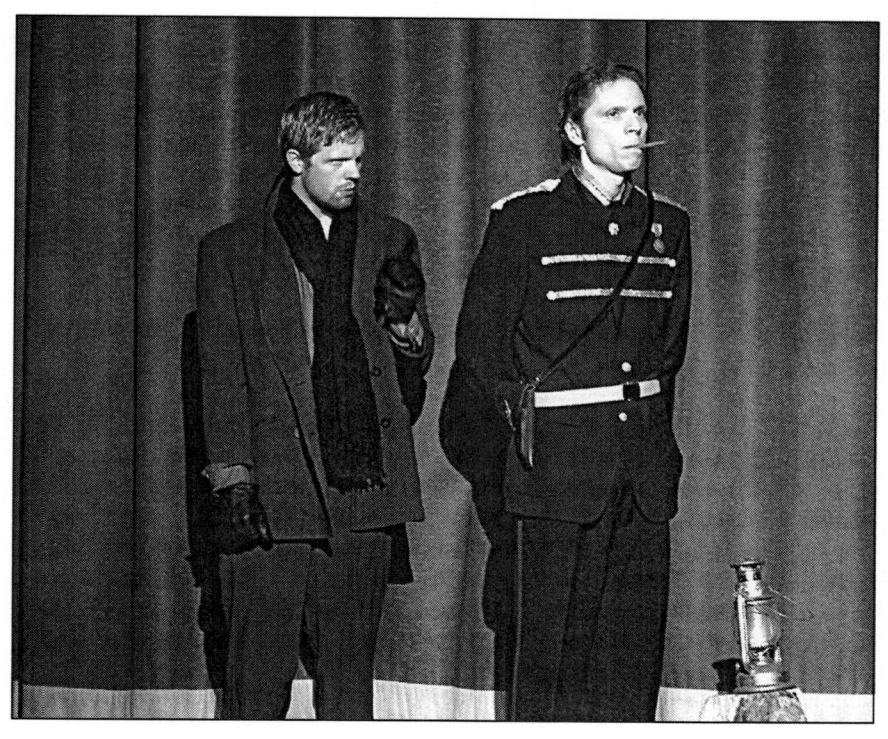

LUCAN (*looking ahead*): Your crude interruption of my morning walk hardly constitutes an audience. Consider yourself lucky. Ordinarily I would have you removed from my path by the scruff of your neck, but today I'll make an exception. You see, in half-hour I too have an audience, one that promises to be tiresome. Perhaps, if I indulge a creature like you, even for an instant, God will credit me this good deed and shorten the impending ordeal. You chose a good day to ambush me. Speak, young butcher.

BENNETT: My Lord, you are in grave danger.

LUCAN (*yawns*): What shocking news. Who is after me this time?

BENNETT: Your own brother-in-law, my lord.

LUCAN: Dear old Jimmy? Who would've imagined? I thought we were getting along so splendidly. Tell me, young butcher, whence do you derive such wild ideas?

BENNETT: My lord, it's true! He's plotting your overthrow as we speak. He had recruited that diabolic doctor, Thomas Grant, who has been on his yacht since yesterday. I do not know what your brother-in-law had promised Grant, but that man has no principles, no honor. He won't think twice before breaking the Oath for his personal benefit. Take my word for it. I've worked under his watch. Sadly, my colleagues do not seem to grasp the full extent of Grant's moral depravity. He had fooled everyone, from the chaplain to Miss Nightingale. She is smitten by him! And the soldiers worship him. It's quite gut-wrenching.

LUCAN (*interrupts Bennett, still looking ahead*): Are you finished, young butcher?

BENNETT: Almost. In light of the situation, I assume that Thomas Grant will not be returning to the hospital corps. Now that he has a new personal benefactor in the face of Lord Cardigan, he will surely abandon his medical responsibilities. The unit will need a new physician. I hope it is not overly presumptuous on my behalf to recommend myself for the vacant position. True, I do not have a diploma from Cambridge, but I am familiar with the patients, their wounds, their conditions. They trust me. And I in turn am bound to them by duty and compassion.

44

LUCAN: In other words, you came to ask for a promotion? Then you should've started with that. You should have said: "Lord Lucan, Thomas Grant is in my way. Please remove him from his post, so I can to slice and dice my patients freely." That would've saved us both a few minutes.

BENNETT: My lord, you are mistaken in regards to my motives. I swear on my life that my primary concern is for your wellbeing – and that of England.

LUCAN (*turns to Bennett abruptly*): Am I expected to believe such declarations? You pitiable gossip boy! If anyone deserves to be removed from his post, it is you! First you interrupt my morning walk, which alone merits court-martial. Then you insult me by suggesting that I have something to fear from my imbecile brother-in-law and that hairy abortionist from Southwark. You truly fathom yourself so significant to imply that I cannot solve a family trifle without your assistance? Back to your victims, butcher!

BENNETT: My lord, you will regret not heeding me.

LUCAN: Out of my sight!

Scene 7

Florence is asleep on the ground in a half-sitting position, wrapped in her shawl, her head on the bench, an extinguished lamp by her side. Grant emerges from the shadow, looking very weak, his every step, every move labored. He kneels near Florence and strokes her forearm. She stirs, raises her head, sees Grant and reels in disbelief.

FLORENCE: What time is it?

GRANT: It appears that I lost my pocket watch. Are you surprised to see me?

Grant lowers himself on the ground next to Florence. Still half-asleep, she stretches her arms towards him, and they embrace.

FLORENCE: I don't understand. I was told that you were sent back to England.

GRANT: Not until all my evil deeds in Crimea are completed. Tell me now: do you like boring tales of political conspiracy?

FLORENCE: If they are told by you – surely.

GRANT: Oh, you're in for such a treat. What if I told you that Cardigan offered me ten thousand pounds to drug Lucan?

Florence shakes her head and laughs after a pause.

GRANT: I know. I couldn't believe it either.

FLORENCE (*suddenly changing tone from amused to hostile*): No, I can't believe that you did not grasp at this opportunity.

GRANT: To stuff my pockets?

FLORENCE: No, to free England from a mid-caliber tyrant!

GRANT: But the Oath...

FLORENCE: The Oath applies to *people*, those illiterate no-names who groan on the surgical table, die of infections and are thrown into a mass grave. Cardigan and Lucan do not belong to that category. Don't you know by now? Some epidemics come in the form of other two-legged creatures that look distressingly human. But we, as medics, must make such distinctions and take necessary actions. Amputate Lucan, as you would a gangrenous limb. By God, Tom, there are no victims on that yacht, only predators of various sizes, all equally despicable.

GRANT: And this is precisely why I cannot bring myself to destroy Lucan. Raglan will replace him with someone even worse. Lord knows, the British army does not lack for incompetent leaders. I simply don't have enough chemicals to drug them all.

FLORENCE (*sighs with embarrassment and looks away*): Forgive me... Mr. Bennett was right – I let the chloroform go to my brain. God, you look abysmal. I suppose, there's no use asking you how you feel.

GRANT: I don't feel much pain, only fatigue.

Florence unbuttons Grant's shirt and presses her ear to his chest.

GRANT (*jokingly*): What do you hear - a requiem for the Famished Bear?

FLORENCE (*straightening up*): What I hear is fluid in your lungs. By God, Tom! How could you have been so negligent? Did you take the medicine I gave you? Naturally, you didn't!

GRANT (*mutters*): I did...

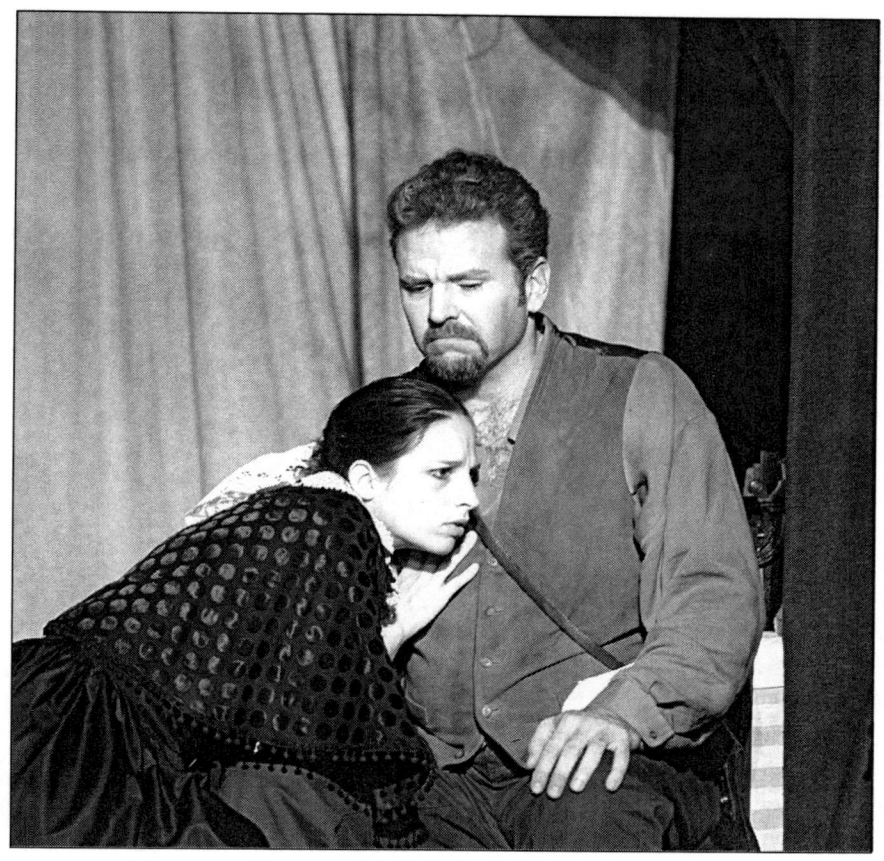

FLORENCE (*not hearing his last statement*): Arrogant fool! You fancy yourself omniscient, immortal... And why should my patients take me seriously, if my own colleague, who sings my praises, dismisses my advice? Well, congratulations, Tom. You have earned yourself a splendid case of pneumonia. What am I to do with you now?

GRANT: Please, sit down. I have something to give to you.

Florence sits down reluctantly, arms crossed, still indignant.

FLORENCE: What is it?

Grant reaches into his pocket and pulls out a yellow journal tied with a rope.

49

GRANT: My intellectual dowry.

Florence shakes her head and pulls back slightly.

FLORENCE: I am not ready to read it. You said it wasn't finished yet.

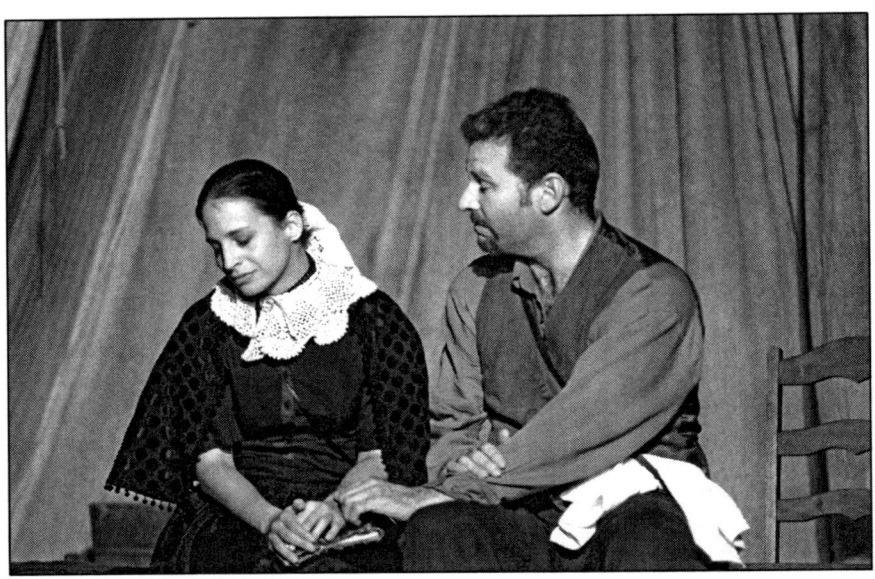

GRANT: I might not have the time to finish it.

FLORENCE: Of course, you'll finish it – upon your return to England! Once this military circus is over, you'll have all the time in the world.

GRANT: I won't be returning to England. We both know it. In a week or two the chaplain will be wrapping me in sailcloth.

FLORENCE: I've had patients in my care recover from pneumonia.

GRANT: How old were those patients? I am no longer twenty... or thirty... or even forty... I have close to five decades of relentless self-abuse. Dear Florence, my body is a museum of horrid habits. It should be donated to Cambridge University.

FLORENCE (*not paying attention*): Very well. Your illness can still be reversed, *if* you surrender yourself to my care.

GRANT: I've outlived many patients, including my own children. This time I shall join them.

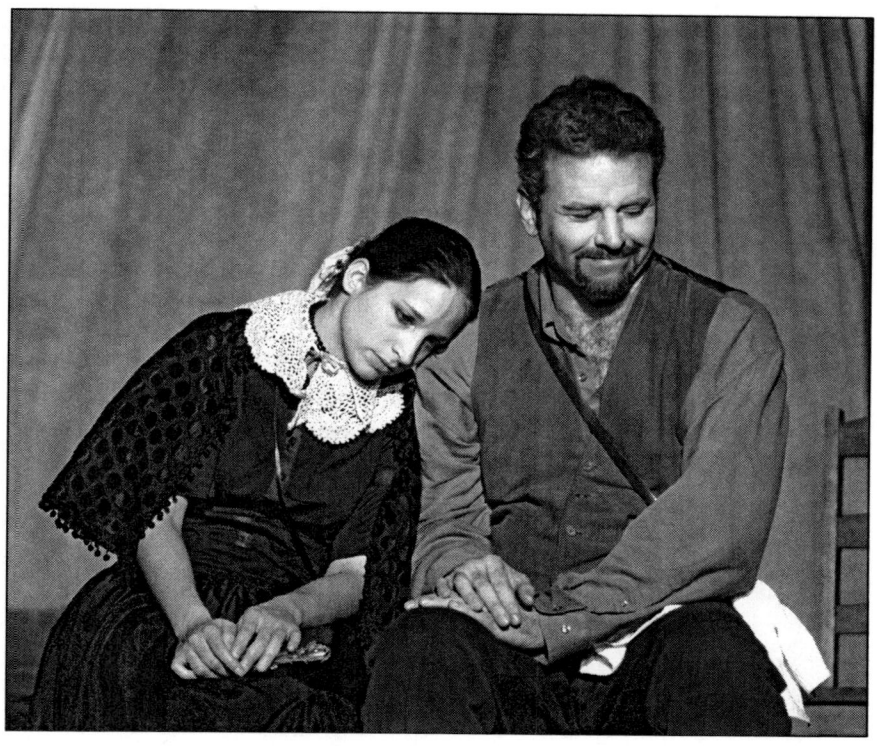

FLORENCE: But Tom, you've had so many opportunities to die, and you've bypassed them all. Why now? What shall I do?

GRANT (*places the journal on her knees*): You shall read over these lines and hear the Famished Bear, growling from the slums of Southwark.

FLORENCE: Don't ruin a perfectly scientific moment with poetic drivel.

Florence leans over and gives Grant a sorrowful kiss.

GRANT: I would not mind prolonging my life just a bit – not for any worthy cause but for my own selfish pleasure.

FLORENCE: Everything we do is for our own selfish pleasure, even the acts that are deemed as noble by onlookers. There is no altruism. There's only vanity that can take so many forms. Behind every lofty cause there is a low motive. I am no better. My mother was right. From the very beginning, I've been indulging my own whims, even while wrapping gauze around bleeding stumps.

Grant shakes his head and laughs weakly.

FLORENCE: What? You find it hard to believe?

GRANT: No, I do believe it. That's why I laugh. It is altogether amusing. First Cardigan offers me ten thousand pounds, and then the unconquerable Florence Nightingale graces me with a kiss. These adventures are worthy of Dickens or Hugo. If you despise lyrical poetry, you must appreciate political satire. (*Looks up and folds his hands jokingly*) Oh please, God, give me another few months. I'm curious to find out how all this ends.

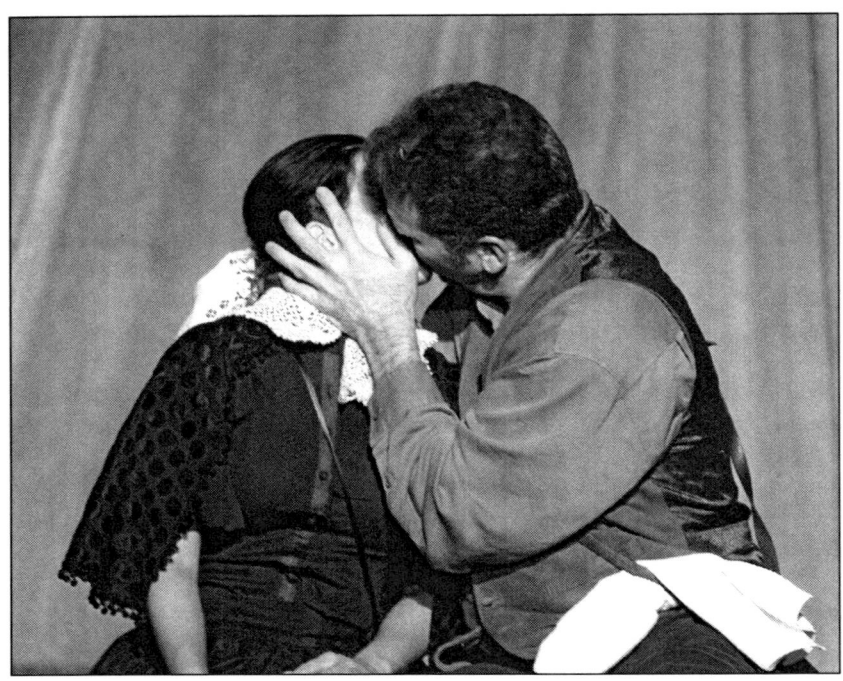

52

They kiss again, this time Grant being the initiator. The kiss is longer and more elaborate.

FLORENCE: Does that mean you will at least try to delay your departure?

GRANT: I promise to obey you if you in turn promise not to marry Sidney Herbert, even if he does become widowed.

FLORENCE: How did Sidney's name surface?

GRANT: His name always hangs in the air, spoken or not. Every tourniquet you apply is dedicated to him. I know it, and it irks me to no end. Be honest: am I hopelessly inferior to Sidney?

FLORENCE (*without hesitation*): Only socially. Not intellectually or even physically. Although, he is younger and better preserved. (*Examines and strokes his face*) Your jaw is every bit as defined as his, and your brow every bit as high. If a man possesses those features, he is handsome already. As a matter of fact, you and Sidney would get along quite well.

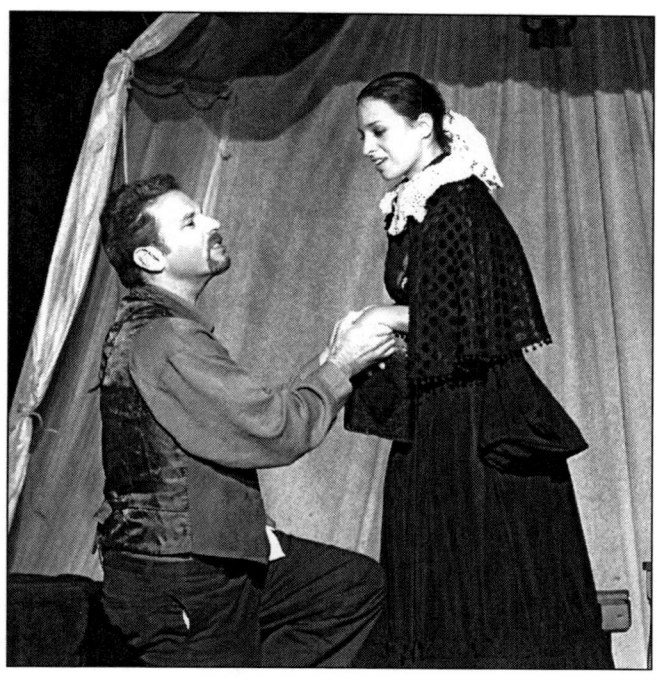

GRANT: You can't expect me to harbor amicable sentiments towards him.

FLORENCE: In Sidney's defense, he is my patron, the one who sent me here. We owe our meeting to him.

GRANT (*without a blink*): Then marry me. Together we'll quake the academia, with or without Cardigan's bribe.

FLORENCE: I suppose, we should go and awaken the chaplain. He must be bored of funerals, poor soul. Surely, he'll welcome a chance to perform a different ceremony.

Florence rises to her feet and helps Grant stand up.

GRANT: We'll celebrate with moldy bread and contaminated water. A splendid feast!

FLORENCE: But there will be no guests. We must keep it a secret.

GRANT: Our secret...

They exit with their arms around each other.

Scene 8

Enter Bennett, dragging Rebecca, whose hair is disheveled and blouse ripped. There are bruise marks on her cheekbones, and her lower lip is bleeding.

BENNETT: What's the matter, Miss Prior? You've turned the hospital corps into a whorehouse, and when I hold you up to your duties, you back down. You are a useless nurse, but apparently, you have other gifts. It would grieve me to see them go to waste.

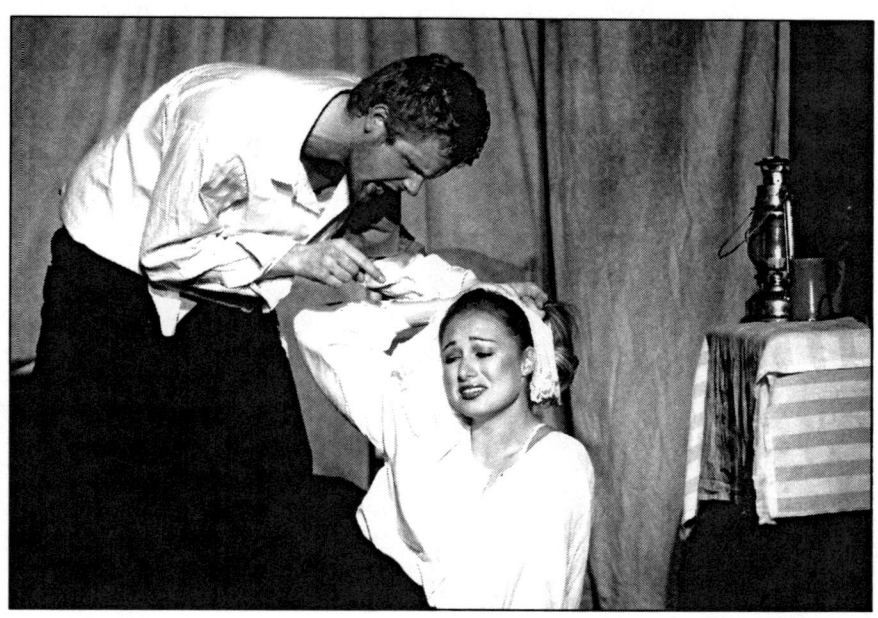

REBECCA (*whining half-audibly*): Please, don't...

BENNETT: Why not? What can I do to you that other men haven't done already?

REBECCA: The God sees...

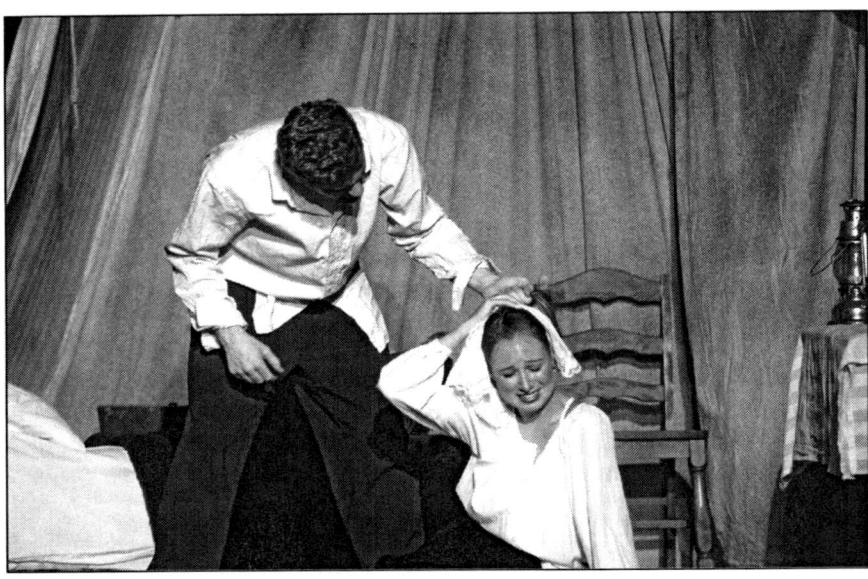

BENNETT: He sees! Why does He only see my transgressions? You still play a virgin with me, even after I catch you half-naked between two drunken soldiers.

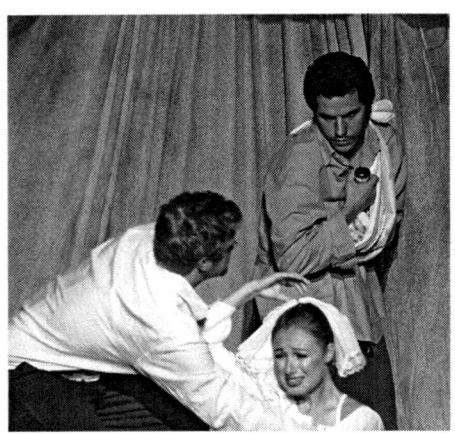

Rebecca whimpers. Bennett wraps her hair around his hand and brings her head close to his.

BENNETT: What? What was that, Miss Prior? Were you about to tell me that the sin of flesh is lesser than that of pride? Perhaps, we should consult the chaplain. What do you think?

56

Martin runs up behind Bennett and stabs him in the back with a scalpel. Bennett releases Rebecca and falls to the ground. Martin stands over him, panting.

BENNETT (*on his side, mocking Martin through his teeth*): Not shabby... You handle a scalpel well. Had I known, I would've trained you as my assistant. I was telling Miss Prior moments ago how I hate to see talent wasted. (*Nods towards Rebecca*) It wouldn't mind sharing her with you. It would be an honor. She can amuse two men at once. It is a proven fact.

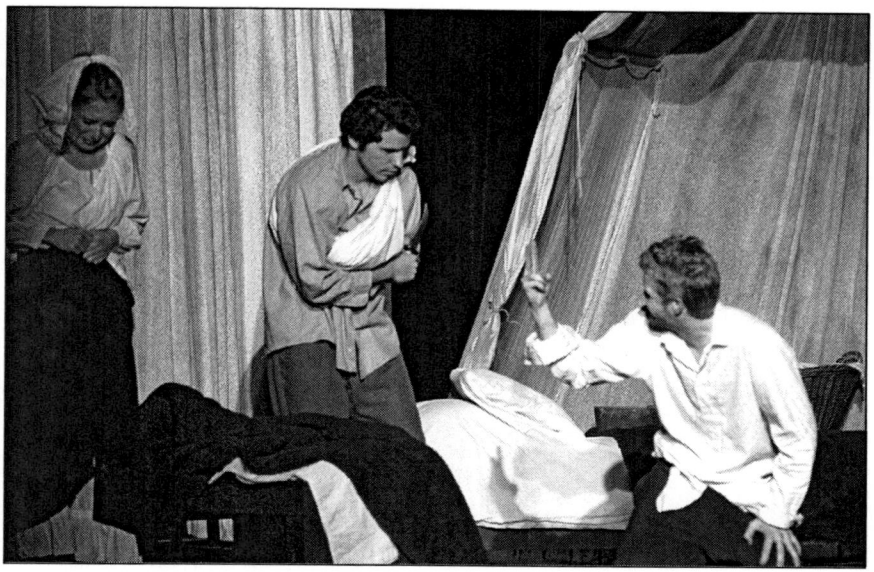

Martin jumps on top of Bennett and plunges the knife into his throat. Bennett's body twitches and freezes. Martin drops the scalpel and runs to Rebecca.

MARTIN: He can't hurt yer now!

Rebecca turns away. Martin squeezes her shoulder. She winces and pulls away.

MARTIN: Look at me! He's dead. The bloody bast'rd... He won't cripple 'nother man, nor will 'e touch 'nother woman. 'Tis all o'er.

Rebecca shakes her head with disgust and keeps backing up.

57

REBECCA: I can't...

Martin drops on his knees and stretches his intact hand towards Rebecca.

MARTIN (*begging*): Don't pull 'way from me. Yer have nothin' to fear. I'm not like 'im. I done many a rotten thin', but I never harmed a woman. I swore to yer I'd be yer vassal 'til the end of me days. Recall that?

Martin remains standing on his knees, hand outstretched, as Rebecca backs away.

Scene 9

Bennett's body is on the ground. Rebecca is in the corner, covering her mouth with her fist. Grant and Florence are standing together, leaning on each other. Martin is on his knees, the stump of his severed hand is out of the sling, tied to the other hand behind his back. Cardigan paces back and forth, desperately trying to look commanding and intimidating. Lucan is observing the scene with contempt and disgust.

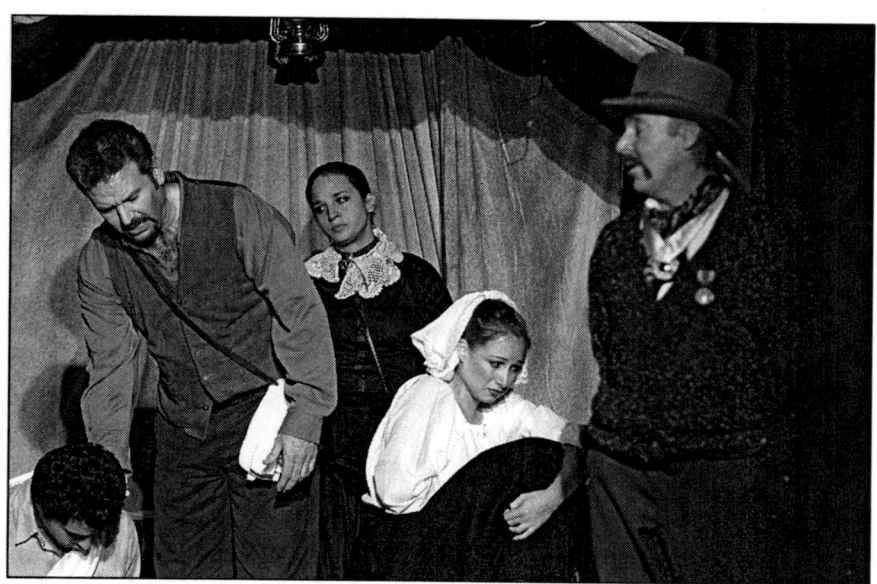

LUCAN: The one-handed thief killed the butcher surgeon. I should've expected something of this sort to happen. It was getting

59

suspiciously quiet at the hospital corps. We were due for a little bloodshed. (*To Cardigan*) Lord Cardigan, what exactly do you intend to do with Private Martin?

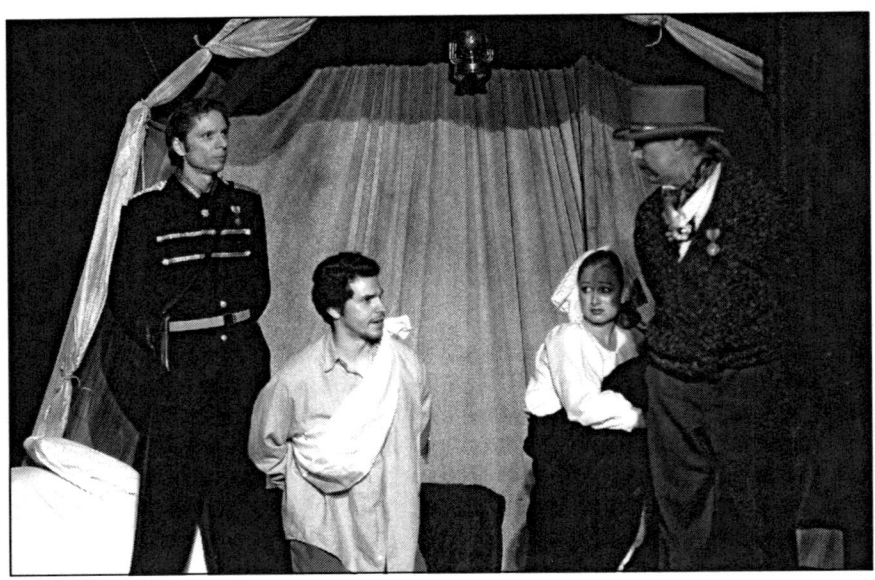

CARDIGAN: He shall receive the same treatment as any other murderer.

Grant steps forward, leaning on Florence's shoulder and panting.

GRANT: In God's name, this man can't be held responsible for his deed. Clearly, he is out of his mind.

CARDIGAN: How peculiar. As far as I recall, it was Private Martin's hand that was injured in the battle, not his head.

GRANT: His head suffered too! Loss of a limb can bring on insanity. Lord Cardigan, listen to me. This is my medical testimony. You can't try Private Martin as you would a healthy man.

CARDIGAN: Dr. Grant, as you recall, I have removed you from your post as a doctor. Your opinion is of no relevance. If I make an exception for Private Martin, what message will it communicate to the entire Light Brigade? Then every soldier will claim insanity as an excuse for insubordination and violent outbursts. He will be executed tonight, as an example to his comrades.

MARTIN (*laughs hoarsely*): Bah! I killed the wrong bast'rd... So many pigs to slaughter, and only one hand...

GRANT: How are we expected to win this war, (*points to Bennett's corpse*) if we have Englishmen killing one another? Family members plotting each other's overthrow...

Grant throws a glance at Cardigan.

CARDIGAN (*nervously*): Dr. Grant, your supervision of the medical unit has proven to be most inefficient. All these atrocities happened on your watch.

FLORENCE (*losing her temper*): Oh, for heaven's sake! Look who's talking about inefficiency!

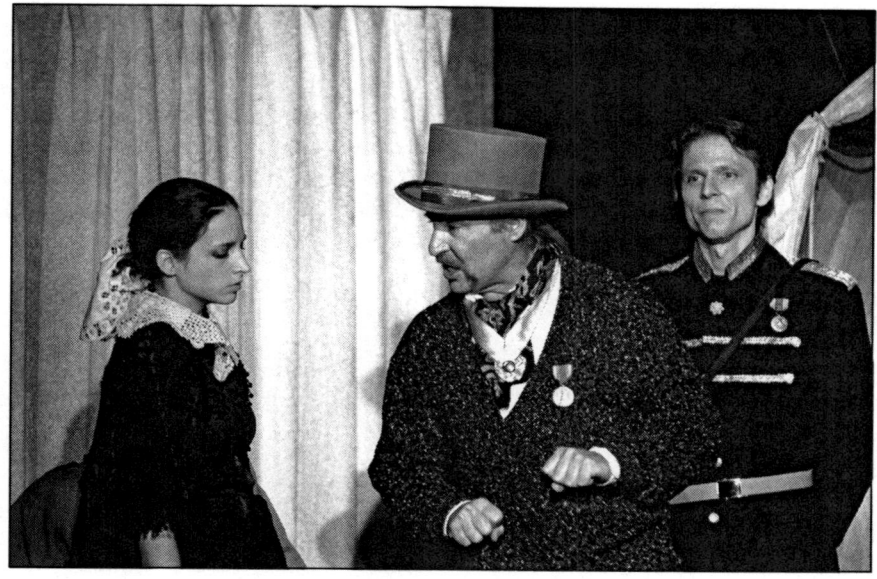

CARDIGAN: Easy, Miss Nightingale. You can dig your dainty little fingers into surgeons and physicians, but please harness your temper with commanders of my rank. Everyone is aware of Sidney Herbert's patronage over you, but even that has its limits. Another outburst on your part and you shall be on the next ship back to

England. Personally, I always thought it imprudent to allow women into a war camp. You may have wrestled your way into medicine, but do not dab into politics. You've already witnessed many things that aren't intended for a lady's eyes.

LUCAN (*to Cardigan, with crude familiarity*): Easy, Jim! Let the mad scientist speak. He started mumbling something about family conspiracy - I'd like to hear the rest. Let him elaborate on that topic before he kicks the bucket. (*To Grant*): Speak as long as you like, Dr. Grant. You have my explicit permission. Nothing you say will be held against you. By the time I come up with an adequate punishment for your audacity, you shall be dead already.

GRANT: I have run out of tirades.

LUCAN (*superficially disappointed*): In that case, does Private Martin have any final wishes?

MARTIN: Yes, yes 'e does. As matt'r of fact, 'e does. A few days 'go, I had my last pinch of t'bacco stolen. Nothin' would please me bett'r than one last cigar, rolled by Miss Prior's lovely hands.

LUCAN (*to Martin*): I like simple men with simple wishes. (*To Rebecca*) Miss Prior, you heard your patient's request. His chivalrous attempt to defend your honor has cost him his life. He'll be executed because of you. Remember that as you roll his cigar. Be sure to tuck the paper in around the corners. It is an art.

REBECCA: I can't. My hands are trembling.

LUCAN: Your hands are always trembling. Now is not the time to be skittish. Imagine that you are working with someone else's hands. When I am overcome by anxiety on the battlefield, I imagine that I am leading someone else's army, not my own.

REBECCA (*gradually regaining composure*): But I don't have any tobacco.

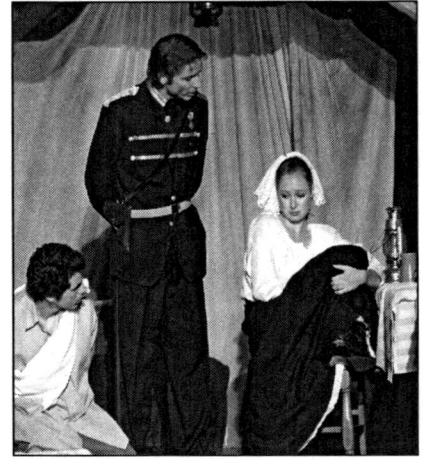

LUCAN (*looks around and claps his hands*): Does anyone here have a pinch of tobacco to spare? (*To Cardigan*): Jim, will you do anything today to justify your existence? Or will you be your usual self? I thought so. (*To Grant*): Good doctor, in your fantastic assortment of chemicals, do you have anything as simple as tobacco? Do you have anything besides rat poison and hallucinogenic substances?

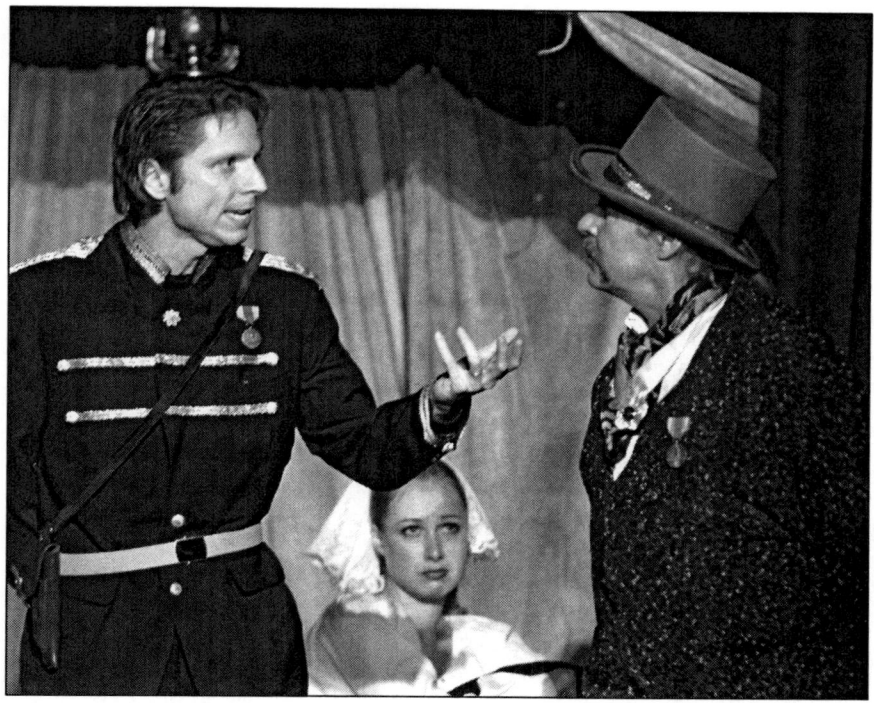

Everyone remains silent. Lucan waits for a few seconds and then throws his arms up in despair.

LUCAN: As usual, I must take leadership into my own hands and sacrifice my own goods! I did not come here to be the star of the spectacle, but you leave me no other choice.

Lucan rummages in his pocket, pulls out a fabric pouch with tobacco and a sheet of paper, then hands them over to Rebecca

LUCAN (*to Rebecca*): Miss Prior, do the honors. (*To Martin*): Young man, this is top quality tobacco, the likes of which you've

63

never smoked. Be sure to savor every puff. Every criminal should be so lucky as to sample such a treat before his execution.

Rebecca sits rolls up the cigar, then walks up to Martin and places the cigar between his teeth with steady hands. Cardigan gestures for Martin to stand up.

CARDIGAN: On your feet! Walk...

Martin struggles to his feet, his eyes on Rebecca. Before departing he glances at her over the shoulder. Martin inhales, preparing to speak; Rebecca raises her hand, commanding silence.

REBECCA (*in a calm voice*): Do not open your mouth. You'll drop your cigar. I worked hard to roll it for you.

Cardigan and Martin exit. Rebecca exits on the opposite side. Grant loses his balance and subsides on the ground; Florence supports him from behind. Lucan stands over them.

LUCAN: I hope you last another hour or two, good doctor. We have too many deaths, and only one chaplain. Now that Mr. Martin has had his final whim satisfied, it is your turn. Ask away. I've already started on a frivolous note, and now I can't stop. What do you wish?

GRANT (*panting and looking Lucan in the eye*): Restore me to my position. I still have enough air in my lungs for a few rounds.

LUCAN: My poor Tom, you have not mastered the art of elegant leisure. This is precisely why you are dying. You have exhausted your nervous system.

FLORENCE (*with bitter sarcasm*): What an astute observation...

LUCAN: When was the last time you ate a three-course meal?

GRANT: Twenty-five years ago, at Lord Middleton's house.

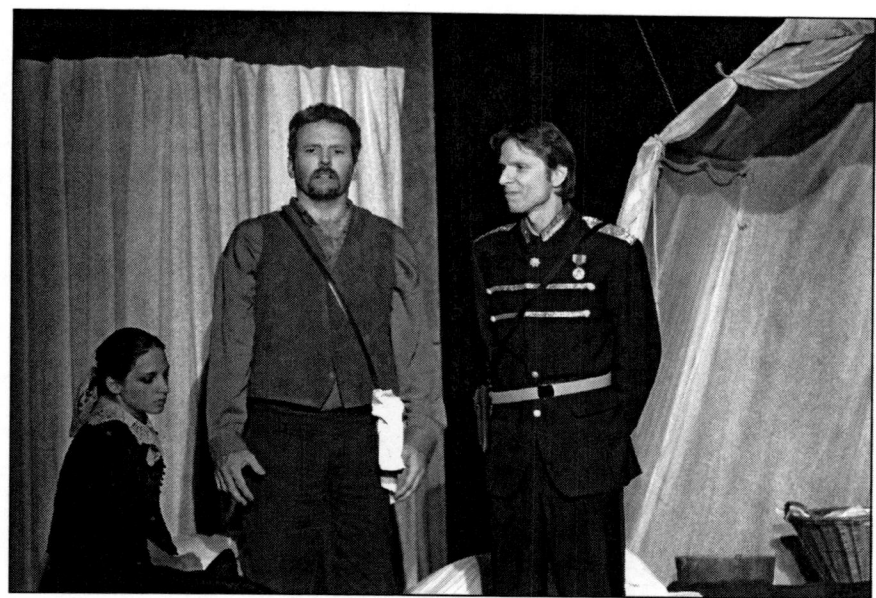

LUCAN: And when was the last time you slept for eight hours without interruption? (*Pats himself on the chest*): Look at <u>me</u>. Would I be as effective a leader if I did not cater to my physical needs? Human body is fickle and frail. Ah, I forgot! You are not human. That's right, you are a bear. Well, do you truly consider yourself a bear, Tom? Bears sleep a fair amount, don't they?

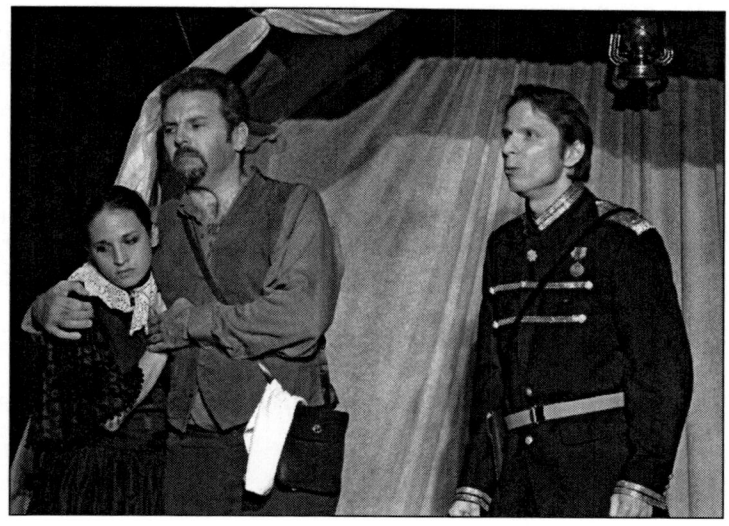

65

FLORENCE (*losing her composure*): For God's sake, stop interrogating Dr. Grant! You've sacrificed a whole pinch of your precious tobacco for Martin and you didn't ask him so many questions. Lord Lucan...

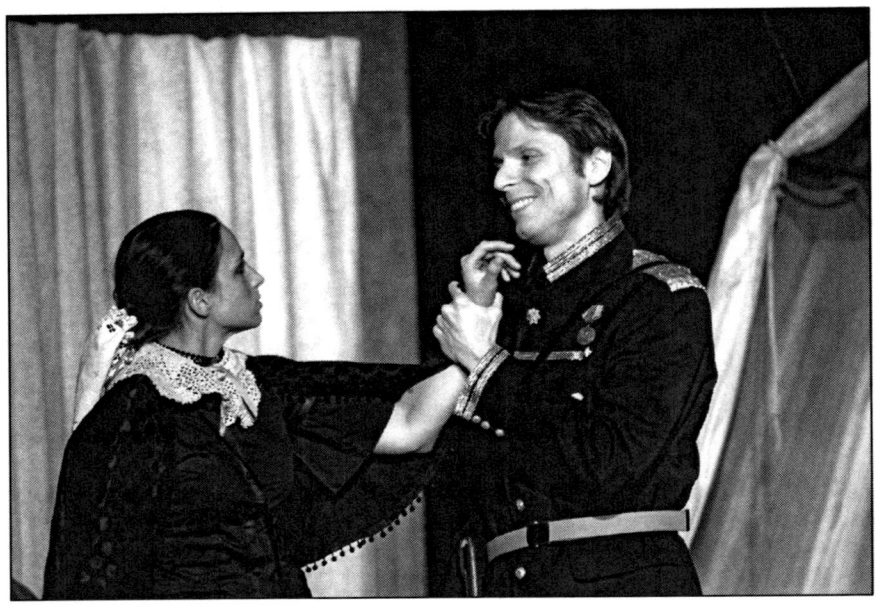

LUCAN: Please, call me George. Unlike my brother-in-law, I do not mind familiarities from a pretty woman, even if she is past her prime. If it will please you, dear Florence, I will honor your lover's request. If he wants to bark bloody mucus all over his patients, who am I to stop him?

Lucan stretches his hand to Grant.

LUCAN: Thomas Henry Grant, doctor of medicine and philosophy, I hereby give you my blessing to resume your dirty and thankless work of which there will be no shortage.

Grant takes Lucan's hand and forces himself on his feet.

LUCAN: Aren't you forgetting something? Here's where you say—

GRANT: God save the Queen?

LUCAN: I would have preferred to hear "God save Lord Lucan", but I suppose, one is never wrong to mention Her Majesty. After all, it was her idea to send us all here. We must thank her for presenting us with this opportunity to show our heroism in such hellish conditions. And if my brother-in-law summons you again, tell him... (*Glances at Florence*) No, I mustn't say such before a lady. By the way, Florence, Sidney Herbert will be thrilled to hear that you have found a new lover. What a relief it will be for him and Elizabeth and their six children.

FLORENCE: I have found more than a lover. Tom is my husband.

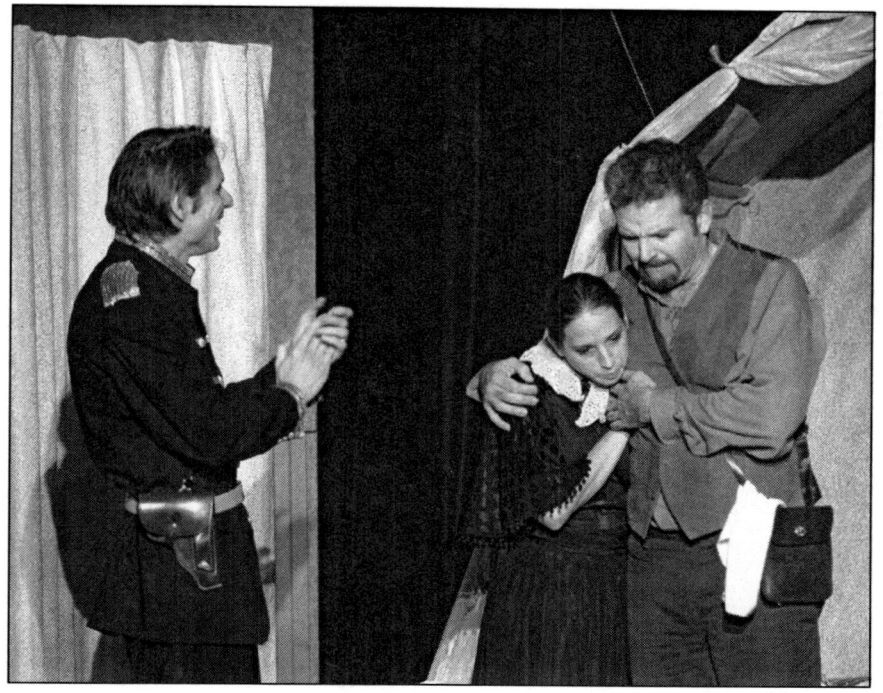

LUCAN: Even better! Why wasn't I invited to the wedding? No matter, I'll be sure to attend Tom's funeral. I shall ask the chaplain to wrap him into something more regal than sailcloth. The British flag, perhaps? That will be my personal gift.

Lucan laughs maliciously. Florence leads Grant away.

67

Scene 10

Florence is sitting alone, clutching Grant's notebook to her chest, an extinguished lamp at her feet. Enter Rebecca, tiptoeing cautiously.

REBECCA: Miss Nightingale, there's much work to be done. The gents are gone.

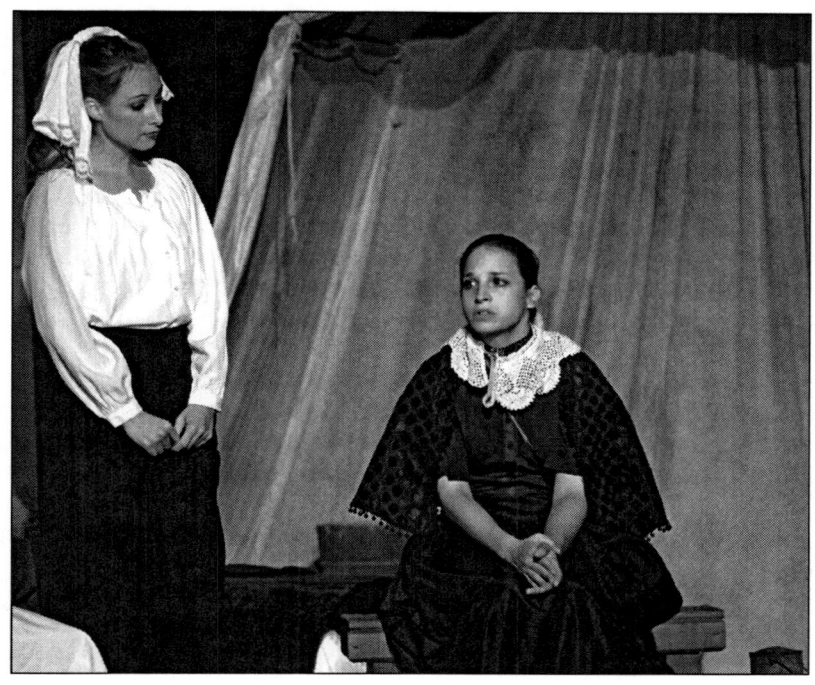

FLORENCE (*expressionlessly*): The gents are gone....

REBECCA (*sighs nostalgically*): Yes, Dr. Grant... (*Cringes*) Mr. Bennett... The chaplain says it will be weeks before the new doctor arrives. It's you and me for now. Surely, we'll have our hands full.

FLORENCE: The gents are gone. (*Laughs like a madwoman*) They are gone!

REBECCA (*draws back tentatively*): Why are you repeating yourself, Miss Nightingale?

FLORENCE: Indeed, why am I repeating myself? (*Turns to Rebecca*) I don't know, Rebecca. Honestly. Nobody is listening, whether I mumble or shout. Young lady, I owe you an apology. I had no business lecturing you on the dangers of premature death. (*Points her finger at Rebecca*) You shall outlive all of us. You'll stand over our mass grave and say: "Fiddle-dee-dee!"

REBECCA: Don't jest like that, Miss Nightingale.

FLORENCE: No, I'm perfectly serious. Girls like you have a guardian angel. There's infinite wisdom in your stupidity. And I have much to learn from you. And you were absolutely right: I was indeed jealous of you, for all the reasons I just mentioned.

REBECCA: Envious, of me?

FLORENCE: I do not grudge you your yellow locks. They are the least of your advantages. It's the hollowness under the locks that I covet. The benefit of being meager and useless is that nobody profits from your death. You may as well be left where you are.

REBECCA: But I don't want to be meager and useless anymore. I want to be grand and famous. No more being cornered by drunken soldiers. Those days are over. I want to receive letters from scientists and generals, have audiences with the queen.

FLORENCE: Is that all you want, dear girl? Don't stifle your ambitions.

REBECCA (*oblivious to Florence's sarcasm*) There's more. I want to have other nurses in my command. (*Ecstatically*) I shall march

70

ahead of them, carrying my own lamp, lighting the way. And everyone around shall bow and say: "Behold: a saint!"

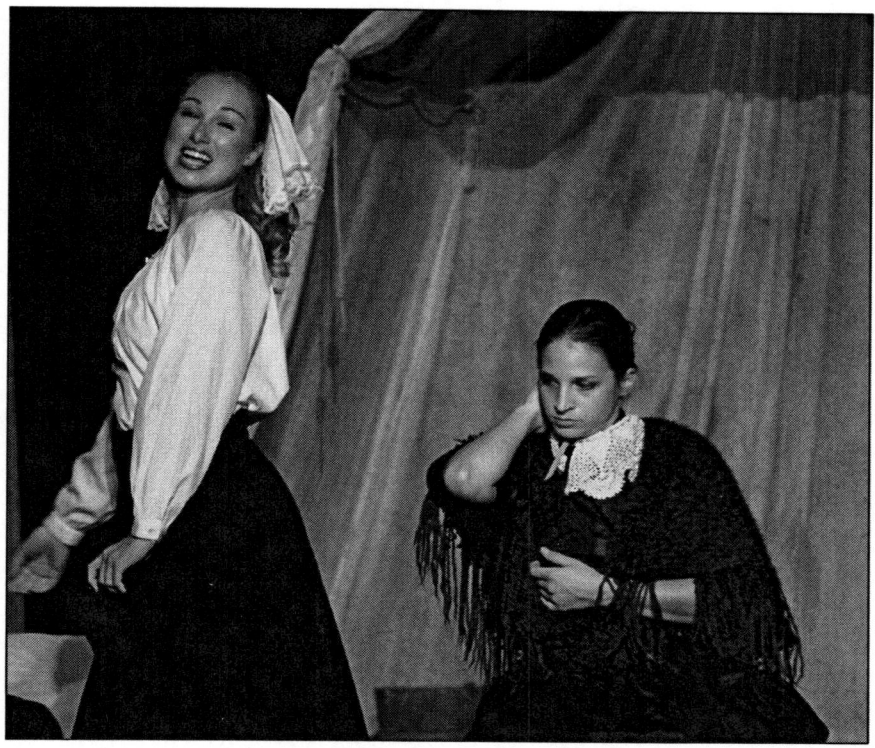

FLORENCE: Your modesty is astounding.

REBECCA: I know! I've promised myself to be humble and modest from now on. No more rouge. No more stuffing gauze into my blouse. Miss Nightingale, you'll be proud to hear that I have ended my friendship with Molly Fields.

FLORENCE: Why?

REBECCA: That friendship was not wholesome for my soul. I need a worthier friend, someone like you.

FLORENCE (*with slight disgust*): Someone like me...

REBECCA: I need someone to teach me how to tie my hair in a bun and scold surgeons when they don't do their job properly. Will you do the honors, Miss Nightingale?

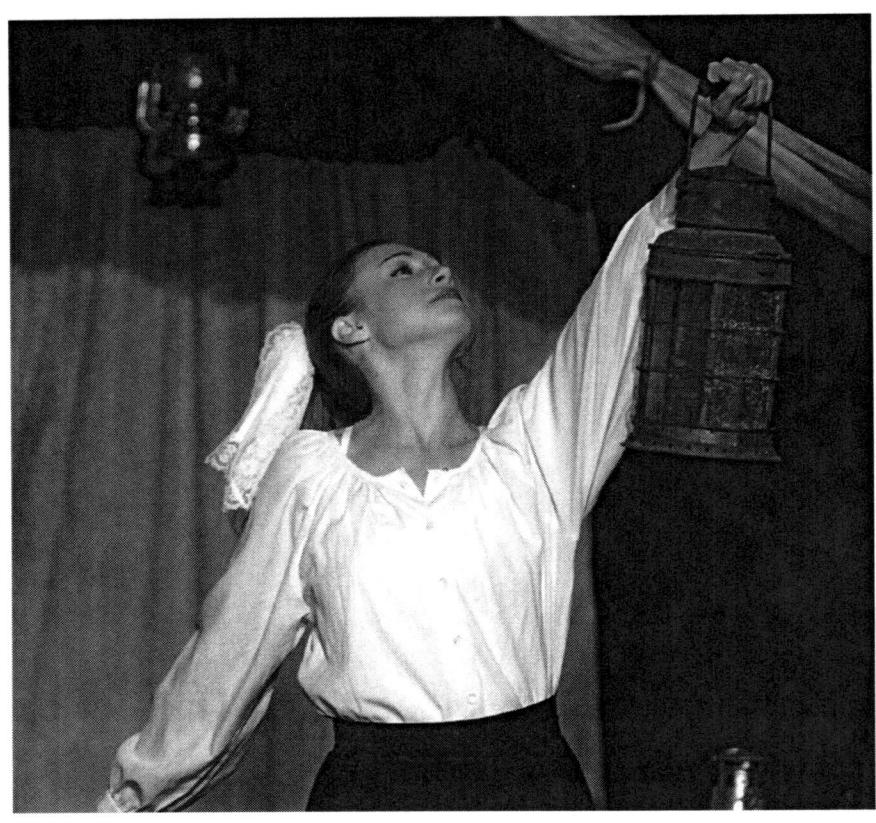

FLORENCE: I could begin by teaching you how to apply a tourniquet.

REBECCA (*reluctantly*): Oh, must I? Is it truly necessary?

FLORENCE: Dear girl, before you start barking orders at others, you will need to learn to carry them out first. This transformation will take time and, as my heart tells me, many more swooning spells.

REBECCA: I am willing to do whatever is necessary. Anything to be the next Lady with the Lamp! But wait, I have more news to share. I have a new gentleman friend.

FLORENCE: Who is the lucky victim?

REBECCA: The chaplain! A future saint needs a godly suitor. Wouldn't you agree? He's been giving me lessons in theology. He's also privy to the latest military scandal. There's talk of Lord Lucan being sent home to England. During his latest audience with Lord Raglan, he had a fit.

Florence puts the vile into her pocket.

REBECCA (*continues*): He started ranting, and cursing, and rolling on the floor. The chaplain was invited to exorcise him. How does the story strike you, Miss Nightingale?

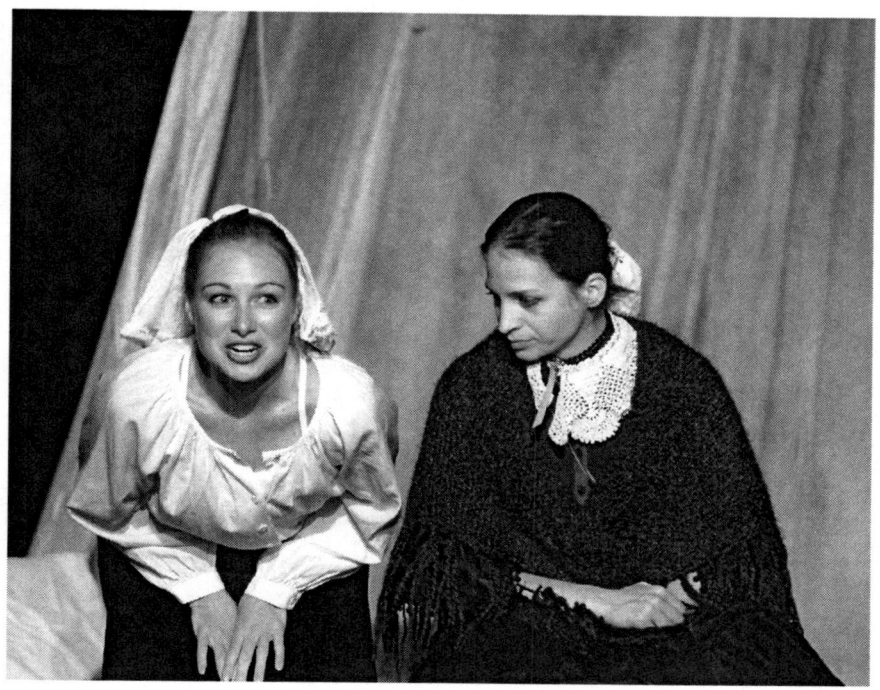

FLORENCE: I am a woman of science. What would I know about demonic possessions or military scandals?

REBECCA: But wait, that's not all. There's a rumor that Lucan's madness was induced, that someone had drugged him.

FLORENCE: Miss Prior, if you are committed to becoming a respectable, graceful, enlightened woman, you must give up the pleasure of spreading rumors. Now go back to your patients. I shall join you shortly.

Rebecca flutters away, self-complacent, leaving Florence to her reverie.

Scene 11

Florence is standing in the spotlight, smiling mischievously and pressing Grant's notebook to her chest.

FLORENCE: My marriage to Thomas Grant that lasted for ten days never made history. Having taunted us about it, Lord Lucan never mentioned it again. He did not even keep his promise to attend Tom's funeral. Early in 1855 Lucan was dispatched back to England in disgrace, to the great pleasure of his brother-in-law, who received a hero's welcome. As much as I begrudged Cardigan his fame, I knew it was only a matter of time before the public would learn the truth about his incompetence. There is nothing more entertaining and gratifying than to see hollow braggarts dethroned. And I had my share of laurel garlands waiting for me in England. What saved me from this atrocious public veneration was a nasty case of Maltese fever which forced me to quarantine myself in a hotel room for several months. By the time I was well enough to reenter the world and resume my work, the madness had settled. And who would greet me at the entrance but Sidney Herbert! Until the end of his days he remained my advocate, my patron, my platonic lover. Thousands of patients have gone through my hands – and thousands more were destined to. Five years after the Crimean campaign, I published a handbook under the most mundane, unimaginative title "Notes on Nursing." Pity, I had to leave out some astute observations and theories. My audience would not reconcile them with the image of the Lady with the Lamp. I still believe that some epidemics come in the form of fellow humans. This is why I did what my husband did not have the heart to do. For now, with a worn-out heart, I stand at the Altar of the murdered men, and while I live, I fight their cause.

75

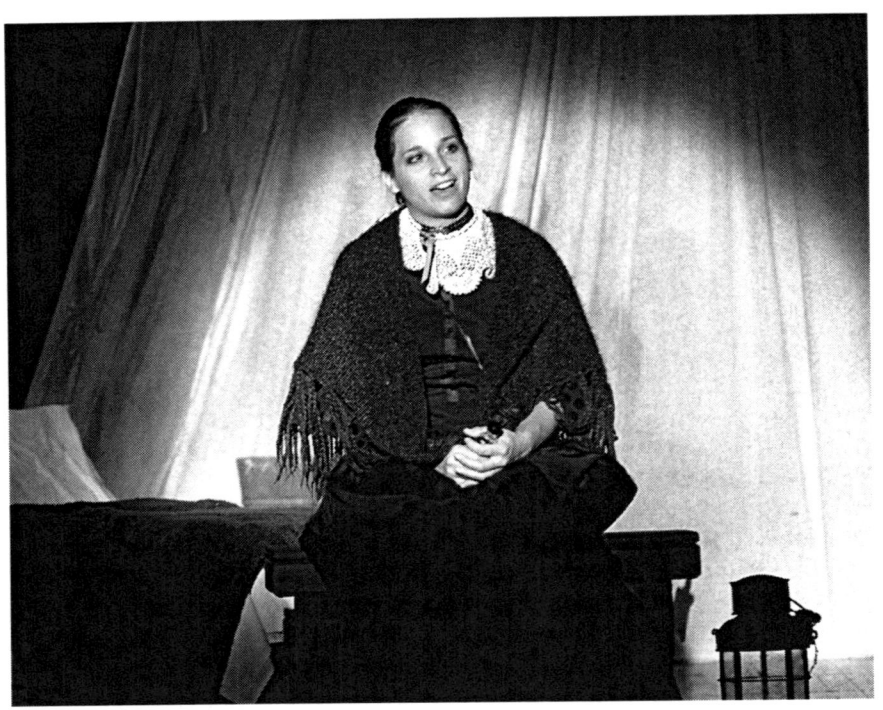

The Lady with a Lamp

About the Author

Marina Julia Neary

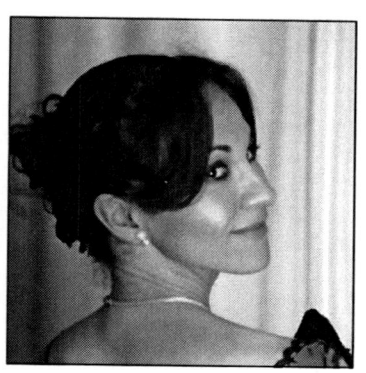

M.J. Neary is an award-winning historical essayist, multilingual arts & entertainment journalist, poet, playwright and actor. Her poetry has appeared in various literary journals such as *Alimentum* and *The Recorder*. She serves on the editorial staff of the *Bewildering Stories Magazine*. Her historical tragicomedy *Hugo in London,* featuring the adventures of the French literary genius in England during the Crimean War, was produced in Greenwich, followed by a sequel, *Lady with a Lamp: An Untold Story of Florence Nightingale.* A specialist on the obscure works of Victor Hugo, she has lectured at the French Alliance.

In 2007 she was commissioned to collect and publish the memoirs of residents from a retirement community in Stamford, CT. The project involved interviewing over forty senior citizens over the age of ninety. A new Connecticut-based leisure publication *Norwalk Beat* has recently brought her on board as a steady contributor. She focuses on the entertainment industry in Connecticut. After having her short story accepted by *Bewildering Stories Magazine*, she was invited to join their editorial staff.

In addition to her writing, Neary has had a career in the performing arts. She has starred in several independent films shot in CT and NY; and, in the 1990s, she competed in various talent pageants in New England.

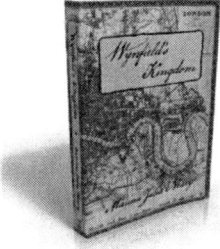

Breinigsville, PA USA
06 December 2009
228707BV00005B/19/P